EPILEPSY EMPOWERMENT

Living an Exceptional Life with Epilepsy

Melinda Curle

Copyright 2014 Melinda Curle

All rights reserved. No part of this book may be reproduced or transmitted in any form or by any means, electronic or mechanical, including photocopying, recording, or by an information storage and retrieval system – with the exception of a reviewer who may quote brief passages in a review to be printed in a newspaper or magazine - without written permission from the publisher.

Perfect Publishing

ISBN-13: 978-1-942688-01-3

Printed in the United States of America.

Dedication

This book is dedicated to all my wonderful friends and fellow epilepsy sufferers. I strongly feel that their lives will be improved and they will find positive engagement and employment if they focus on what they can do and create win-win situations in their lives.

Table of Contents

Acknowledgments................................. vii
1. A Devastating Diagnosis 1
2. Awakening.......................................7
3. Epilepsy Empowerment....................... 11
4. Conquering the Fear........................... 21
5. An Abundance Mentality 27
6. Increasing Self Esteem 35
7. Habits to Stop NOW 45
8. Open Your Heart............................... 51
9. Create Your Own Support Team................. 59
10. Build Your Offensive Line 65
11. Tapping into Your Creative Side................ 71
12. Raising Your Value 79
13. Workplace Environments 87
14. A Home-Based Income 91
15. Passive Income Creation 101
16. Heroes 109
17. My Story...................................... 119
18. Resources.................................... 127
19. About the Author 139

Acknowledgments

I would like to acknowledge the wonderful friends that I have in the staff and students at Fairfax High School and Lanier Middle School for encouraging me to follow my passion of becoming a writer. Some of them have been incredibly helpful in bringing this to light and encouraging me to do a book launch. Many of them have helped me to see how a positive attitude can turn things around and encourage success.

I would like to acknowledge the wonderful friends and family who donated to my kickstarter campaign. My awesome cousin, Barry McClure, my mother, Sally Curle and the wonderful Facebook friend, Steve Christenson.

I want to thank the Epilepsy Foundation and the neurologists in the medical profession for helping to make the lives of people with epilepsy more comfortable.

A Devastating Diagnosis

The 15 year old had been looking forward to this day all week. She did not know it was the last day she would ever think of herself as normal again. She and her mother were going shopping for a dress for her first "real" dance at the high school, and this was the day. As they walked into the store, she felt a strange tingling at the tips of her fingers and feet, and barely noticed it; when she did, she shrugged it off as excitement because of the occasion. As her mother talked with the owner of the boutique in the small retail center in what could have been Anywhere, USA, but was really just outside of Macon, Georgia, the tingling in her arms and legs, which had gotten stronger, grew to the "pins and needles" of a foot that had fallen asleep. The girl, having first thought it excitement, felt the first creep of fear enter her body like a real creature, her neck suddenly began twitching uncontrollably. She could tell that something was wrong. A pounding in her ears grew to a crescendo, her vision narrowed and grew dark around the edges. Fear washed over her for a few brief seconds. As the neurons in her head fired off at random and the terror gripped her, she tried to scream, but it was lost, the seizure hit her full force, a bulldozer plowing over a flower. Consciousness stopped as her body was wracked with convulsions.

She awakened to find herself lying on a gurney in an ambulance. The next thing that she remembered was the EMTs telling her "You experienced a seizure." They kept looking at her with a mixture of care and concern on their faces. When they arrived at the emergency room, the staff tested her vitals, drew some blood and monitored her level of consciousness. After she had stabilized and they felt she was fine, the resident suggested the family take the child to the Pediatrician, and a battery of tests ensued over the next four months. The seizures – that's what they now knew they were- kept coming. They would be gone for a week, ten days, then three days in a row would be racked with numbness, blackouts, high speed rides to the hospital as the mother, unable to deal with a child who had a medical condition, demanded answers from doctors and nurses who struggled to find answers that "more tests" were sure sniff out. The answers were short, and were not answers. Allergies. Hormones. Mental health. Drug abuse. All were bandied around as a possible reason for the seizures. Each one came back negative, each one led to even more foolhardy theories.

"Your daughter has epilepsy." This was reported by the new Neurologist one day, at the office of the fourth specialist the family had visited, this time at a well-known hospital in Atlanta. He was tall, dark haired, and reported the information the same way he might have described the score of a football game he did not care to watch. The girl's ears perked up, not knowing what epilepsy was, and was quietly terrified when her mother began crying and her father cursed under his breath.

While the doctor may have struggled with his bedside manner, he spent the next hour explaining what Medical Science knew about Epilepsy – quite a lot, actually. They still didn't know the Why, but they knew a whole lot about the How. It was a central nervous system disorder that affected nerve activity in the brain; basically, he said, the brain of the epilepsy sufferer simply could not process all the electricity it produced and at times, this resulted in a short circuit which manifested in a seizure. Each patient experiences it differently, but many seizures can be classified into a range of categories. It was a life sentence, but one that could be controlled through anticonvulsants. There had been successes in the surgical field, but those were out at the very edge and the research was still very new. At the end of the conversation, the girl had hope, her parents did not. A very visible wall had gone up around the mother, and a different wall around the father.

The coming weeks and months saw the mother negating any after school activities, as though the teenager, who had been a bit of a tomboy, was suddenly made of glass. The father chased down the family attorney to get the girl on any kind of disability benefit she could qualify for. After the first year, when the Social Security Disability Income began, she was now officially labeled a "person with epilepsy". Kids she had known since Kindergarten now avoided her. Several times, she tried to explain what it was, and the explanation fell on deaf ears. The avoidance was the worst. It seemed like they didn't know what to say to her.

Her grades gradually decreased as her medication increased. Her self-esteem suffered. The anticonvulsants worked, usually; but they were expensive, and the team of doctors her father had recruited were constantly increasing the medication, and eventually adding a second. She lived in fear of The Big One, that gigantic Grand Mal that would knock her out and kill her when the convulsions couldn't be stopped in time to prevent some weird accident. She tried to push it out of her mind that the grand mal seizures could take her life. At doctor's appointments her parents monopolized the conversations with the doctor because of their own fear of having a daughter with epilepsy and somehow that meant that she need not be involved in the conversation that concerned her. The girl was not discouraged from asking, she just couldn't get a word in edgewise.

When she was sixteen, her mother forbid her to get an after school job, and since she had epilepsy, she could not get a driver's license. At 18, she got her first job, but quickly learned that due to the disability income, she could not work more than 25 hours a week. Her parents decided that she couldn't go away to a college, she needed to study locally at a community college, since, of course, she was a "person with epilepsy" and somehow, having a seizure locally was better than one elsewhere. And after all, her mother was quick to point out, her family had sacrificed so much for her; expensive medications, doctor visits, and such, why would she want to go away for college? She would never be able to work, the Social Security would provide for her. She shouldn't be so selfish, the family had suffered for her, and she should think of her little brother, he was healthy, certainly not a person with epilepsy like her and he would be needing to go to college, too.

This young lady faced, nearly every day, the mental and physical stigma of her diagnosis. As a result, a misunderstanding about what is occurring and the reactions of others to a seizure began to influence her own attitudes and reactions. However, they don't have to! She made the decision to train herself to become a positive person despite those who told her to "know her role" and you are going to learn how to do that as well. You can minimize the psychological damage that epilepsy causes since those seizure episodes trigger a fear response in not only the person who had them, but the people who you rely on; friends, family, and acquaintances. We tend to like life to be predictable and seizures throw a wrench in our plans. However, we choose our responses to stimuli. We are capable of choosing a positive response to seizures. The diagnosis of epilepsy can be devastating in its implications but it is not the end of life. In fact, many wonderful people with epilepsy are leading extraordinary lives.

It is important to understand that while parents are well-meaning when making medical decisions for children and teenagers, it is disempowering to the individual. They start to believe that other people know better and their opinion of their own care isn't worth as much. I started going to doctors at the age of 13 myself. I was embarrassed that my health was discussed between my parents and my doctor. However, it was a necessary evil. It took a while as an adult to empower myself and realize that I had control over the decisions regarding my health, and as I learned more about health and fitness, my quality of life grew exponentially. As I have talked and interacted with others who have epilepsy, I have come to realize that we can all grow and empower ourselves and live the life that we want; it is there for the taking.

Awakening

At its core, Epilepsy is simply a neurological disorder that affects nerve cell activity in the brain, leading to seizures. The causes are still being understood, but at the root of the issue, it is a short circuit in the brain seemingly driven by too much electricity in the neurons. After a seizure and a period of rest, the sufferer is usually none the worse for wear, although post-seizure symptoms include fatigue, headache, and localized weakness. There are often bumps, bruises and a bitten tongue. However, the majority of seizures are not life threatening.

The larger issue at play in this work, is the psychological issues that serve to prevent those with Epilepsy from leading healthy, productive lives. In a study published in the British Medical Journal by M. Floyd and associates, people who suffer from epileptic seizures also suffer psychologically as a result of them. Feelings of self-worth and doubt closely follow fears of simply having another seizure. More than 69% have concerns and apprehensions about employability. Moreover, these psychological effects are compounded by the number of seizures an individual has undergone, the severity of them, and the time between each event. The study brings to the forefront what should be intuitive, people are judged, incorrectly, for the disorder, not the individual. When sufferers become the symptom, they can cease to lead productive and engaging lives.

This fear may be more intense when you are away from home and people may be completely unaware of your ailment. This stems from the fact that when you suffer a seizure, most people stare unbelievably and gawk. They are typically caught off guard and don't know what is happening or what to do. That cannot cripple your lifestyle as your seizure isn't under your control and it doesn't harm anyone except yourself sometimes. With ever increasing awareness about epilepsy, this is bound to pass, though your confidence cannot lie in someone else's behavior, only in yours.

Why Me?

The initial days after a diagnosis are filled with feelings of despair. This feeling is all too real to anyone with a chronic disease, but, with time, and with concepts I put forth in this book, we will see that this is a natural process that may take a while to overcome, but it can done. It is so important to realize at this stage that there are many more people out there who struggle with the diagnosis and feel the same way. Do not shy away from how you feel, rest assured, you can have and lead a normal life, but you will have to create it. I will help to show that if you can be positive, you can find the success you want. The first step in leading a normal life is realizing that you ARE normal, with a controllable medical condition. Labeling yourself an "epileptic" or a "person with epilepsy" gives the condition more importance in your life than it deserves. You are a thinking, loving, caring, talented human being who braves neurological seizures from time to time. The real question is a simpler one. Can you lead a normal life? This is the one that will decide whether this disorder will break you or free you. Make no mistake, between concerned loved ones that think you are fragile, potential employers who think that hiring you would be a mistake, and the general public that don't have a clue what it is but are scared of it, you are now treading water in the deep end of the pool. I am a living testimony to the fact than you can! I have spent years making the mistakes that this book shows you how to move easily past, but the truth still boils down to one thing; YOU have to make the decision to want to succeed. No person, no book, and no friend can do that.

Once you realize that even the questions and apprehensions that run in your mind are mirrored in the minds of others with similar conditions, you can begin to realize that you need to take the next big step in your life, that of empowerment. We are going to spend a lot of time on that idea and the ways that you can embrace them. The structure of this book is driven by the fact that if you are not mentally and physically prepared to be successful, you cannot go and build a business or a career. We are going to build up your mind and your physical body, then we are going to show you a variety of ways to look at a career. You may be perfectly happy in the one you have now, but as you grow and empower yourself to think big again, you may realize there are options that you never saw because you and the people you trusted may have been taught to think small and safe.

So let's start on getting you back to believing in you and looking at the ways to make sure you have all the success you deserve!

Epilepsy Empowerment

"Incredible change happens in your life when you decide to take control of what you do have power over instead of craving control over what you don't"
–Steve Mariboli
"Life, the Truth, and Being Free"

Empowerment is believing in yourself and that you have the ability to take control of the course of your life. It is understandable for someone who has experienced a seizure, or loss of control over their body, to feel that they have lost control over their life. When a person does not feel empowered, they may have low self-esteem, feel unmotivated to set or go after goals, and cease working towards happiness in their lives. You can empower yourself through emotional and physical activities that get you more in touch with how you affect your environment.

It cannot be stressed enough that even though you have epilepsy, you are a very, very important person with a lot to offer the world. Your set of challenges, with epilepsy, is, of course, different than other people, but it is no deterrent to you being wildly successful. It is so important for you to tap into your creativity, to focus on the positives in your life, and to focus on the things that are you are good at and that you can do. It will go a long way towards improving your quality of life as well as the satisfaction you gain at work. Too often, we interface with doctors, employers, and well intentioned loved ones who can only point out what we cannot do and try to force that belief into our minds. This can be very discouraging and many people can slip into depression because of the negativity and the focus on the limitations imparted on them from the people they love and trust. Negativity does not empower you, nor does it define you.

A great place to start is to keep a journal of seizures. When they hit, how long before they passed, and how long was the recovery. Take that and put it in the context of all the available hours in a day, a week, a month, a year. A lifetime! Right there, on the printed page, in your handwriting, is proof that the seizures are brief. They are a tiny fraction of the time that you are living. I know recovery can be uncomfortable, and can take some time, especially when well-meaning bystanders call emergency services and you spend the next four hours in an emergency room waiting for the "all clear" that you already know you have, but this still should not stop you from taking charge in your life and the time you are not directly dealing with a seizure. The more productive you are, the more joy you will discover. Not only that, but as you seek to improve your health and become more creative, you will learn to naturally control your seizures and, with improved seizure control, you will sculpt a more fulfilling life. The journal can start this trail of success by showing the patterns of the seizures. Record health changes that you make and monitor the increase or decrease in seizure patterns. This will give you a better idea of a lifestyle that works for your own seizure control.

This book is written to help focus you on creating this wonderful life and to find purpose in that life to live it more fully. Many people don't realize that the limitations that we place on ourselves are just that – SELF imposed. Events such as seizures can induce fear into our lives for no positive gain. When you eliminate this fear of seizures and the excuses that come with a chronic illness, you can see all that you are able to accomplish. Not only do you become more valuable in the workplace, you will learn to enjoy life to the fullest and you will end up making more money. All your positive actions will add to that feeling of power and creativity.

Tapping into your creativity will help you uncover options for making money and employment paths all around you. Soon you will start to recognize that there are lots of trails and methods of earning to be sought out, not just a 40 hour week in a cubicle for a pittance. You may even find a career path in the suggestions in this book that is perfect for your situation. In the process, you will discover that you are a powerful person who just happens to have epilepsy. You can positively impact the world.

I'm speaking from experience. I have had, many, many jobs. I have lost or been laid off from many jobs. My seizures were probably an indirect reason for the termination, but at the same time, I had not taken the time to understand my weaknesses created by the seizure disorder. I lived in denial about my seizures and the medication's impact on my performance for a long time. This led to being much less efficient at jobs, thus creating negativity from me and the people who employed me. After being fired from yet another job, one year I sought out a neuropsychologist. She performed a series of tests and discovered that I was weak in processing speed. This made me uncompetitive in many jobs. Despite my love of meeting and talking to people in person or on the phone answering questions, as hard as I tried, gathering information was difficult and I could not retain the information that was exchanged during the conversations. This was a weak area for me and it was going to take a long time to become proficient enough for the job.

Employers don't want to take years to train someone to simply be competent. They need that employee up and running efficiently very quickly. Once I understood my weaknesses, I began targeting jobs that were more suited to my strengths.

A breakthrough for me was when I began to target job markets that involved opportunities and things I was passionate about. I have loved swimming since I was a little girl and didn't stop swimming when I was diagnosed with epilepsy. I never feared it, and as a teenager, I was on swim teams and reveled in the competition. There were a couple of times that I had a seizure in the water and my coach had to pull me out. Even though logic would tell all of us that I could easily drown during one of these incidents, it did not stop me from swimming. I made known that I had random seizures, those people with me were aware of it, and I refused to let fear cripple that love that I had of the competition and the water. Of course, my coaches required that my mother be on deck in case anything happened, but she was willing to make that sacrifice for me.

Recognizing that swimming was one of my passions enabled me to utilize my knowledge and teach other people to swim. I started out as a volunteer for the Adaptive Aquatics program at Oak Mar Recreation Center in Oakton, Virginia. The management recognized my commitment and I was quickly hired as an instructor part-time. This was a wonderful experience for me. Not only was I in water which was a great joy for me, but I was helping other people with disabilities to learn how to appreciate swimming as a recreational sport. I never let my epilepsy hold me back in the years I was a swim instructor.

Another job I felt particularly positive about was substitute teaching at Lanier Middle School. I had tried my hand at teaching and discovered that dealing with parents, juggling curriculum presentations, and classroom management was very difficult for me due to the slower mental processing due to my anticonvulsants.

After two years of discipline problems with students, I determined that maybe my ideal teaching environment was one on one with students rather than in large groups. I traded a full time teaching position for tutoring and the less profitable but less stressful substitute teaching path. Taking this step backwards in my teaching career helped me to learn better discipline skills and better aligned me personally for success. I still actively substitute at Lanier and it has a wonderful staff that has helped me tremendously. I have found a spot in many of the teacher's hearts as I willingly fill in for them and follow their lesson plans.

A few years ago, I did indeed have a seizure at Lanier. It was in the middle of a break, while eating lunch. The staff, very accommodating, took great care of me, and then simply went on about their business. The next day, they asked for some additional emergency contact numbers, but they did not make a big deal about it. I was still a teacher and they were concerned about my well-being. It was only later that I found out they had actually put me on the preferred substitute list despite the seizure and that was why I had been getting more and more requests to substitute at Lanier. I was and continue to be very grateful for the opportunity that I have had to interact with such a positive staff and to continue my learning with them. Whenever I am there, I try to make sure to be friendly, engaged, and helpful in whatever way I can.

A life with epilepsy does not mean a small life. History is filled with men and women that have managed epilepsy and not been affected by it. Julius Caesar is one of those great humans who was not conquered by epilepsy. The tales his exploits that have come down through history are many, but his brilliant tactics, his leadership, and his self-confidence are all underlying parts of the great story of his life.

In his Life of Julius Caesar, Plutarch of Chaeronea tells us that while still a general in the Roman army, Caesar was captured by

Sicilian pirates in the Mediterranean Sea. When the ransom was set at 20 talents of gold, Caesar burst out laughing and told them they should ask for much more, perhaps 50 talents. The pirates sent word of Caesar's capture and set the ransom at 50 talents of gold (3550 Pounds). In the ensuing 38 days before the gold was collected and the ransom paid from Miletus, Caesar acted more as victor than captor, mocking the pirates and their leaders, telling them directly that he would hunt them down upon his release, and upon being released, collected a fleet, attacked the pirates, and had them put to death at Pergamon, exactly as he had told the pirates he would do. The side story to this is that the Roman politicians turned a blind eye to the pirates in the area, since they offered these senators bribes. Thus Caesar not only was striking out at the pirates who had captured and ransomed him, he was lashing out at the entire Roman political machine, a trend that continued through the rest of his life as General and then Emperor of Rome. It would seem a foolish thought to believe that Caesar "suffered" from epilepsy, in fact, it would be more likely that he never even thought of it at all.

We can all embrace this self-confidence, especially when we achieve success in something. Focusing on the things that you are good at not only empowers you, it can be even more beneficial for someone who struggles with epilepsy. By concentrating on your success and what you do well in life on a daily basis it will help you raise that self-worth and increase your control of your destiny. When someone struggles with seizure control, it can take a toll on their own feelings of self-worth and detract from that confidence. You must not fall into the pattern of focusing on the limitations that the well-meaning doctor, the family, and friends try to place on you. The government gets in on it, too, restricting military service, vehicular operation, or even the amount of work that can be done to someone suffering from seizures who also receives a disability benefit. The medication that you take is also going to rob strength from you- side effects can relieve you of productive time, sleep, and energy as well as slowing down your mental processing ability or causing drowsiness, the costs of the medication can be prohibitive, and not covered under an insurance plan since it is a pre-existing condition. For some people, the side effects of the cure are to build a new set of limitations in the mind that the cause never did.

Now, the logical place to worry about this empowerment is "outside". We make changes to our environment, friends, jobs, even locations. What if I was to tell you that a great deal of the positive change that we need is right there between your ears? Mark Waldman is a neurological researcher who in the last two decades, has crafted (some say proved) several amazing theories about brain development and our responses as individuals to outside stimuli. He is the author of several books, most notably, How God Changes Your Brain, and has used brain scan technology to look at faith, at its most fundamental level, that of simply a positive role in a person's life. His motto is "Change your brain, change your life." His research has proven that optimism is the best way to exercise your brain. He has stated that our current psychotherapy lacks this optimism, because it simply dwells on the idea that "here's your problem, here's your solution," and the therapist never asks you, 'What are all the wonderful things going on in your life?' By using positive thoughts and a gratitude journal for as little as seven days, the brain begins to physically change. After 3 months, the changes are profound. His ideas on a demonstration of faith (in positive outcomes) through meditation for as little as 12 minutes a day, concentrating on those positive things in our lives, begin to show physical changes in our brain structure that can be seen in brain scans.

Research into negative thinking has shown that all thoughts begin in the prefrontal cortex of the brain, no matter whether those thoughts are good or bad. The positive ones arrive from the left, the negative arrive from the right. Every three of those positive thoughts is negated by the arrival of just one negative thought. Waldman has thus recommended that you keep five positive to one negative. How? Thought suppression. In actually watching brain activity while the subject was "thinking" positive thoughts, brain activity in the negative right prefrontal cortex slowed and then shut down altogether.

Of course, sometimes you just can't get the negative out of your head, and then, the research has shown that a person can simply understand thoughts as "outcomes" instead of "bad". Our brains cannot determine a fantasy from a reality, so by mentally limiting the ideas as good or bad, we begin to control other emotions tied to that thought process. Take driving, for example. For those of us with seizures, an event while driving could be catastrophic. We fear it. Logic and chance tell us that the odds of it happening are very slim, in most cases, but the fear of it happening can overpower that logic, even if we have never had a seizure while driving. A child has never seen a boogeyman under the bed, yet they are still scared of it and worry about it every night while trying to go to sleep. The most important part to realize is that your worries, doubts, and fears are false. You are concerned about them happening in the future, but in many cases, they have never occurred in the past. Understandably, when we look at Post-Traumatic-Stress Disorder, where individuals have had a tremendous amount of negative experiences in their past, we know how that can affect their view of the future. Flashbacks during certain phases of sleep can be common, since the brain is not being actively managed by the conscious mind. A great many things can be learned from Waldman's research, and that is the empowering part of it.

This is where the positive aspect of the research comes in. Rely on what you do know! If you have chosen not to drive, then being worried about having a seizure while driving is an absolute waste of time. The control of our environment, then the reassurance of positive thoughts to overshadow the negative, can dramatically change our view, indeed, the actual makeup of the brain. Every "negative" image the brain sees or visualizes actually releases a neurochemical. Obviously, if we can limit that release, we begin to change.

Long before I met or became aware of Mark Waldman, I had begun to research and drive myself to a positive belief structure. I felt that positive thoughts contributed to a positive lifestyle. I quit focusing on weaknesses and began to focus on the positives and my health improved and my ability to control my seizures improved. I simply looked at it logically. The more I thought about it, the more I realized that the bad things just weren't likely to happen. Negativity can be detrimental to your health.

The challenge of this is that the human brain is designed to give more importance to negative thoughts than positive thoughts. This can be traced back to our evolution and the idea stems from needing the ability to forecast what might happen. Thousands of years ago, and even today in some remote places, you had to worry about being attacked and eaten by a wild animal. You had to go source your food on a daily basis. Thus the brain learned to develop a sort of "worst case scenario" based on the information it received. The ability to envision ideas ahead of time, to forecast what could happen, allowed to plan against those potentially negative outcomes. The real end result was that it drove the development of civilization. Don't want to get attacked and eaten? Build a dwelling. Want to ensure food for the family and in the future? Develop agriculture and domesticate animals. Don't want to have a seizure at work? Ah, I caught you! That is an example of a negative thought that you are forecasting and should not be a primary focus. Of course you should have a plan for what to do if you have a seizure event at work, but it should not be seen as a negative thought, merely a planning opportunity. Unfortunately, the same reason that we were able to be successful as a species can be the limiting factor holding you as a person with epilepsy back.

This negativity can manifest itself as a phobia, but not in the grand sense that we generally give the word. We all know people who are scared of flying, yet have no issue riding in a car. Many of those same people have had or been involved in a car wreck, yet they still think of the car ride as safe. They have never, not once, been involved in a plane crash, yet to them, it is not as safe as the car ride that they personally know is dangerous. The facts tell us that there is one plane crash for every 20,000 flights. The odds are amazingly low that you will ever get in a plane crash. Yet there is that person in our group of friends that is terrified of the plane flight. Here is where the idea of actually documenting the frequency of your seizures comes in and showing yourself that the amount of time dealing with a seizure event is tiny compared to the time spent living a life. Do not let a minor series of events shape your life!

Mr. Waldman and his doctrine, Neurowisdom, is listed in our resources section, and I cannot help but say that, since I arrived at many of his same conclusions in a completely different manner, his ideas on positive thought and faith are just short of amazing and they are very worthy of note in your own research about empowerment.

Never forget that there are many ways for a person with epilepsy to be successful and find happiness in their own lives. The key is to remember that your life is different and will require a certain amount of additional (or different) effort than the person who doesn't have the same issues, but the potential reward is an amazing life that you can engage in with pride and a feeling of fulfillment others can never grasp.

Conquering the Fear

"One of the greatest discoveries a person makes, one of their great surprises, is to find they can do what they were afraid they couldn't do."
–Henry Ford

One of the strongest men on recent history, Theodore Roosevelt, suffered from severe epilepsy, a bad eye, and asthma. Roosevelt, known for his hard "cowboy" personality and his bravery in the Spanish-American War, became President of the United States at age 42. Before and after his political career, he continued in his personal drive to be a great naturalist, soldier, historian, author, and world traveler. He not only conquered his fears, he proved to the world that epilepsy was merely a medical problem that need not cripple someone; you can continue to charge ahead with your own steely determination and fear nothing.

Fear holds people back from achieving and accomplishing things that they may want regardless of whether they have epilepsy or not. People become focused on what could happen, and the output of that fear is many times stronger than the input. For someone who has experienced a seizure, it is a reality that they may have another one and that one could be at work, thus jeopardizing their employment. For the vast majority, this fear is unsubstantiated, since over 75% of those with epilepsy control it with medication. The majority of the time, they will not experience a seizure event. Yet they spend huge volumes of energy worrying to no positive effect about "what if" instead of using productive energy to focus on family, career, or a healthy lifestyle.

So how do you face this fear? Face the problem! Look at the worst case scenario and decide how you will deal with it. The idea that you shouldn't go hiking because you could have a seizure and fall off a cliff is silly. You should absolutely go hiking, but stay away from the extremely steep areas of the mountain if it that important to you. That idea probably is foolish for 99% of us, but I guarantee it is an excuse for someone. An excuse, not a reason. Quit dealing in excuses, start dealing with reasons! Quit overanalyzing the problem! Watch out for thoughts that are rooted in fear. Choose your solution based on what you know, not what you fear. Select a positive thought to replace foolish or unfounded fears. Stand up, change positions, physically move to a different spot in the room … all these things can help you shift your mind to a more positive state. Not only will this technique reduce your fear, it is a great way to retrain your mind and think more positively – actively filling your mind with positive images. This exercise is a simple way to reduce the amount of negativity going on in your head by forcing focus off of the silly and zooming in on the practical.

Look to embrace where you are right now. Accept this as a baseline for your health, both mental and physical. Accept today as a baseline for your employability. Accept that you have some fears, but you are now working on overcoming them. You cannot go forward from here until you know, honestly, where here is. When you have sought these answers, and been honest with yourself, you can embrace you for your strengths and weaknesses, and begin the road to improvement. Denial will keep you right where you are right now. Underemployed, unhappy, and underwhelming.

Uh-oh. I said it, didn't I? UNDERemployed. "But I have seizures and they will fire me if I have one." No they won't. You have legal protections and your employer does not want to get involved in a wrongful termination lawsuit. Once again, it is fear, not actual seizures that are holding people back from finding and keeping a wonderful job. Perhaps no one ever took the time to build value in the individual, or perhaps they only told them it couldn't be done. Once again, the active elimination of fear is essential to success on the job. It will free your mind to focus on your work. With that renewed focus, the epilepsy sufferer will be able to engage more in the workplace. The release of the fear will help drive creativity and productivity. When you begin to focus on the positive things in life, you are not focused on the negative impact of a seizure. That positive mental attitude breeds goodwill with employers, as they want employees that are positive and engaged. They want to have an environment that is uplifting and cheerful; happy employees are productive employees. Concentrating on your own health issues is not profitable for an employer and neither is it productive for you. It is absolutely a habit you can break!

Your mind is a powerful tool and when it sends the message to you that you can't do something, you probably won't even try. Many people believe they cannot have a certain job because of their seizures, or that certain jobs will increase the frequency of seizure events. They are right. You are not going to be a pilot. You cannot be a truck driver. But each of these industries have dozens if not hundreds of associated positions acting to keep the plane in the air and the truck going down the road. An awful lot of the behind-the-scenes jobs in these industries pay more than the more illustrious job we coveted. There are many industries that offer flexible schedules and less stressful environments for the employee who has epilepsy. As you release the fear you have been programmed to feel, you owe it to yourself to understand these positions.

Think of the real effects of your seizures and medications, look to your seizure log we have discussed and find patterns in your life. This information helps to transform your fear into information, and that can be used to drive your success. Take action and live positively!

You can become stuck in a rut when you let yourself believe that you can't work due to the impact of the seizures. I have certainly been there! Many times during my twenties, my seizures were unpredictable, and I felt hopeless. I could not understand the mental and medical side effects that were going on and how important it is to focus on your strengths rather than trying to muddle through. Even when I undertook jobs that were supposedly easy, if it required multitasking, I was dead in the water. I was stuck in a rut and not looking like a very good employee because of my slower processing speed and the drowsiness from the anticonvulsant that I used. A smarter thing to do would have been to look at the things I was good at or enjoyed and follow that trail to a more enjoyable career.

It took years for me to understand the concept of focusing on my strengths, having a positive attitude, and taking the steps to improve myself EVERY SINGLE DAY. For a long time I assumed I was doing a good job since I was doing the best I could, but I would not seek feedback from my employers that could help me be better. I knew I was slower than my co-workers at certain tasks, but it took a neurologist and some simple tests to help me to recognize that I needed to focus on my strengths. This doctor wisely pointed out several potential career options, such as medical billing, that could engage me at a pace and place that was good for me. It was not exactly my dream job, but it was something that I could do with the combination of seizures and high intellect that was me. I had to learn to manage a different set of distractions, and do plenty of double-checking for accuracy, but I could do it at my own pace and a break-through seizure was not cause for alarm.

So identify your strengths and identify your passion. Focusing on your strengths shifts your mind to a more positive mentality. Identifying your passion gives you more purpose in life and diminishes the time wasted thinking about fears. Later on, we are going to talk about ways to monetize those strengths and passions, and creating passive income. In this book, I will introduce different ways to earn an income that will not require you to be dependent on transportation.

Take steps to improve your overall health. It has been proven that actively trying to improve your general health will improve your seizure control. By being proactive about your health, you will also reduce the anxiety you face with your seizures. Sooner or later, your doctor will tell you that your condition is idiopathic and they really don't know what is causing the seizures. They do know that there are thousands of things that can cause them, but the actual trigger? It may well be that only you can figure that out. The unknown is so much more troubling than the known when it comes to life in general; it is even more so when it comes to seizures.

> *"Nothing in life is to be feared. It is only to be understood."*
> **–Marie Curie**

Heavy metals can cause seizures. Do a heavy metal cleanse. No, don't listen to rock music turned all the way up. There are a variety of products and diets on the market that can help you to remove harmful metals, such as lead and mercury, from your body. Educate yourself! Google the "water cure" and understand the relationship to dehydration and brain dysfunction. This was one of the best things I ever did in regards to my personal health. Find out how much water you need to drink and make that part of your health program. Make sure that you take sea salt with the water to replace the minerals lost by high water consumption. Eliminate processed foods from your diet. Get lots of exercise. Simple steps such as these help to eliminate the fear of having seizures by helping to eliminate the secondary causes of some seizures. By being proactive, you will be exerting positive control in your life, maybe for the first time since you were diagnosed. The positive feelings this brings on begets a snowball effect in other aspects of your life. Waiting for the next drug or the next appointment to be the miracle cure requires other people. Other people may care about you, but they may have dozens of other concerns besides you. Being proactive chips away at that fear and helps your brain focus on the positive.

An Abundance Mentality

By now, you have probably thought I have lost my mind. I haven't. I have changed mine, though. What changed? I realized that all too often, we look at the glass as half empty or half full. I finally came to see that the problem is usually that there is too much glass. What changed? I got tired of being the poor little girl with epilepsy. I became active in my treatment of the disorder, I became reinvigorated about my life. I studied many ideas and in some ways, Stephen R. Covey summed up my feelings after I had studied many philosophies and life tenets for over a decade. Abundance Mentality.

> *"People with a scarcity mentality tend to see everything in terms of win-lose. There is only so much; and if someone else has it, that means there will be less for me. The more principle-centered we become, the more we develop an abundance mentality, the more we are genuinely happy for the successes, well-being, achievements, recognition, and good fortune of other people. We believe their success adds to … rather than detracts from … our lives."*
> –Stephen R. Covey

I had finally realized that the world is full of potential. There is more money in the world than I could spend, more people than I could ever meet, more ways to empower myself than a lifetime of empowerment study could reveal to me. In short, I adopted an Abundance Mentality. The Epilepsy Foundation is still actively looking for a cure for epilepsy in Western medicine, but there are volumes of ways that epilepsy has been viewed and treated in the societies of the Far East. In short, I realized that if all I ever tried to do was to manage my current state of health and finances along the same way we are traditionally taught in the United States, I was setting myself up for disappointment. When I saw the abundance out there, I realized that if I opened up my mind and used my creativity, I could have a more amazing and empowered life with or without epilepsy.

This abundance mentality showed me that there will always be new opportunities and chances. The person adhering to a scarcity mentality suffers the pain of worry that there is never enough. This pressure manifests itself through pressures that they will somehow only get one shot. If that shot is not in the bullseye, then you have failed. To the person with the abundance mentality, if they miss – a target, a sale, a goal, they just reload and shoot again. No worries. This drives to higher performance since with it, you operate under less pressure an anxiety within your own mind.

Often I share with people that they can change their lives. They hold on to the belief that their doctor is the one with all the answers and the next prescription will be the one that finally controls the seizure. They tell me holistic healing isn't an option for them. This is a scarcity mindset. There are many things that doctors don't understand and cannot explain. This is where the handful of medications come in. At times, the doctor is just trying to find something or a combination of prescriptions that might work. There are many healthy lifestyle choices that a person can make that don't require a prescription and will still cure and heal chronic illnesses and lead to seizure control. Help yourself and educate yourself! As you do so, you will feel more empowered about your own health.

Opportunities to improve every area of your life are all around. It is that old friend and enemy, the mind that places limits on what we believe we can do. Much of the time people only attempt things that they think they will be good at. They look at some traditional method of doing something and determine whether they will be able to do it. Take transportation, for example. The vast majority of Americans get from place to place by driving a personal vehicle. When that is not an option, you must look to taxi services, buses, bicycles, walking or a subway to get places. Finding alternatives to transportation via a personal vehicle is easy. Asking friends for a ride becomes easier the more you do it; the key is to have plenty of people in your sphere of influence that can help, and to remember who is doing who a favor. Offer to pay for gas, buy a coffee or lunch, or simply say "thank you" and mean it.

Just as you clean a home, you need to keep your mind clean of the hints of a scarcity mentality. When you see those thoughts and ideas creeping in, broom them aside and throw them out with the rubbish! Don't be too serious. You may think that the sky will fall if you fail, but it won't. The sun will come up, the rain will stop. You need to remind yourself that very few individual moments will matter in the course of a lifetime. How that life is lived will matter much more. When you start worrying more about the moment than the concept, you become overly nervous about the wrong thing and POOF! You have just welcomed failure back into your life as a guest and it is the new obstacle in your path to success. If it's a game, you might now fumble the ball. If it's an exam, then you may not study or sleep well and you may now fail the test. If it's a date, you may come across as needy or aloof and not as your usual, more relaxed self. Regain your empowerment by remembering all the opportunities you have been afforded and know that it is part of a river of chances flowing constantly through your life.

Focus on that abundance, not on the lack of it. What you focus on, you will be able to find in abundance in your world. Since you can't take in everything around you, your reticular activation system- the focus system in your mind- will bring into focus where you focus your thoughts. This will allow you to see the abundance around you right now. If, for instance, you are struggling with money, don't focus on the lack of it. Focus and think about the abundance of it and the myriad of ways to make money in the world today. As you begin to shift the negative to the positive, you will see ideas and opportunities "pop up" to make your scarcity an abundance. You didn't see them before because you were not in the correct frame of mind to notice them.

A great example of this was a friend of mine who is a writer. He basically can do anything that involves the English language – articles, novels, copy, you name it, and he does it. The downside was that he had hit a slow spot. He was struggling to find enough jobs and simply pay his bills, much less be anything approaching successful. Instead of complaining, he refocused his efforts on his schedule and on the little work he had to do. When the phone began ringing, he was there ready for the work that came in, not curled up on the couch having a pity party. To this day, he keeps that same schedule. Up at six a.m., in the office by eight, and he usually stays in it until at least six p.m. He focuses on the abundance of what he has and the rest takes care of itself, because he is inadvertently networking new business through driving his current business and he is "tuned" to hear when someone needs a writing project done.

A big key to cultivating an abundance mentality is showing your appreciation. Appreciate the things that you do have. You may not have the best of health, or the greatest job, but you are actively taking the steps to improve them both. The old adage of the man with no shoes complaining about his lot in life until he sees the man with no feet is appropriate here, but our abundance mentality encourages us to seek to help the other guy, too. Picking up someone else when they are down is not only the right thing to do, it is a sign that you have begun to realize that there is an abundance out there and you are willing to share it. You must appreciate everything in your life – food, family, home, friends, and so on. This not only helps your mood daily, it helps others see things that they perhaps had not thought of. It can also help you notice things that you may have missed or forgotten about. That "good vibe" within you helps drive success, however you define it. Make a habit of appreciating something in your life, even if you can only start with a few minutes each day.

Another aspect of this shift in mentality is to get organized. Some of the negativity may simply be caused from not feeling good about your life in general; how many times have you or a friend started off a bad day with lost keys? It just seems to go downhill from there until you finally collapse in bed muttering about how terrible things are. Yet if you were organized, you would have known where your keys were, you wouldn't have been hurried to get and then spill the coffee, you wouldn't have missed the bus, you would've been on time to work, etc… Have your home clean, your clothes folded, your digital files in place, and your finances organized. "A place for everything and everything in its place" is where you start. Years ago, and I cannot remember where I read it, a study was done among people suffering from depression. Researchers found that just 30 minutes of light cleaning and organizing by a patient had a profound impact on the mood of the individual. They felt like they had done something and they had something tangible to show for it. Hold yourself to a higher level of order and discipline and you will see results in creating the abundance mentality.

Seek out and change the negative aspects inputting themselves in your life. If you get a scarcity vibe from media and television (that is what advertisers get paid to do), think about what you watch or learn to pay no attention to advertising hype. Seek out news channels or programs that give the facts and don't editorialize them, record your favorite shows and fast forward through commercials. Or just cut down on the amount of television and media that you watch or read.

I'm going to get in trouble for this part, but replace the negative people in your life. We all have that friend whose entire life is a train wreck; limit the time you spend with them. They are not helping you or themselves with their negativity, so don't let them bring you down. If having coffee with Sandy leaves you feeling depressed because her life is a dumpster fire, limit the number of coffees you have with her, or have the coffee and then tell her you have an appointment or a call to make. Even better, level with her and say that you are done with scarcity and negativity, she needs to be, too. You may find that Sandy craves having a pity party for herself. Find and befriend a different person that has an abundance mentality. Unfortunately, Sandy is a cancer for you. Unfortunately, you may work with a whole lot of "Sandys" and you may have to decide that the whole company or industry is wrong for you. We will get into that later in the book, but right now, remember that rebuilding you may require finding a lot of "new" in your life. You cannot BE an enabler, nor can you HAVE an enabler.

This reinvention of your network of friends may also extend to you support group. Many times, I have seen epilepsy support meetings descend into a long string of complaints about doctors, medications, insurance, life, driving, family, etc… This is certainly the venue for this, surrounded by people that have similar issues, but take it upon yourself to be the leader and optimist in the group. Actively steer the discussion away from negatives, discuss the abundance mentality, bring other people into the idea of what you are doing and get them on board. If one person can make a difference, imagine the power of 10 or 100! If you cannot change them, then seek out another group. Some groups just have a different "feel" than others, due to tradition, economics, and a myriad of other reasons. Rebuild your group or become part of one that embraces the abundance, not the scarcity.

Think of it this way. Your family, your church, your friends; they are all in a sort of constant stable state, no matter how messed up or dysfunctional that state may be. You sit in the same pew each week. You watch the same shows from the same chair. If you can drive, you park in roughly the same place every day, be it work or the grocery store. When you begin to change things that change can start to affect those around you, because they may take it as a sort of weird declaration that things just aren't good enough. I've been told that I don't "act right", whatever that means, simply because I was tired of being sick. Well-meaning friends and family can try to bring you down, because they have been taught to believe that you are somehow fragile. This is not just because you have epilepsy, it may simply be because you are trying to be healthier, or finish school, or write a book. When my first book Seizure Free was published, I had an acquaintance who I thought was a friend tell me that I was a danger to the community because I was encouraging people to try holistic healing. I never understood why until I began to realize that to her, nobody but a doctor should prescribe medication or recommend an alternative healing method. This was someone that I considered a friend, yet here they were, bringing me down, cheapening my value somehow because it didn't seem right that I should have a voice in the healing community. So keep an open mind for these sorts of things as you go forward with the changes in your life. It may hurt. A lot. People you love may not understand why you are doing the things you are doing. Keep them positive by being the positive role model, but understand that they may not be ready to see you change. You will, of course, but remember that we are all in each other's lives to change them or to be changed. You can be the positive one and show them how good life can be.

That change will also mean that you should look for other positives in print or online. Read, listen, and watch personal development material. Besides reading your favorite personal development blogs, read success stories in books and magazines. These will help you to drive positive relationships with a new group of people in life, business, and health. Now share this knowledge! Don't hoard it. If you feel like there isn't enough of something, give some of that thing away. This is a great way to acknowledge how much you have. Do you feel like you are not making enough money? Donate some of what you do have. Not enough love? Show that there is by giving it away. Not enough validation, appreciation, recognition? Give it all away. It's hard for something to seem scarce when you're giving it away.

When you do this, you are creating win-win situations. People with a scarcity mentality tend to see every relationship in terms of win-lose – "It's either me or you, buddy, and I want it to be me." People with an abundance mentality, on the other hand, try to create mutually beneficial relationships where both parties can win. Instead of winning an argument, for example, try to reach a consensus that you can both be happy with. Instead of competing, collaborate.

Increasing Self Esteem

"To establish true self-esteem, we must concentrate on our successes and forget about the failures and the negatives in our lives'"
–Dennis Waitley

The logical outcome of the abundance mentality is the increase you have in your self-esteem. You must have worth before someone will pay you. In this, your self-esteem becomes an integral part of your success on the job and, more importantly, in life. Building self-esteem for someone who has a seizure disorder is important since low self-esteem may make you less likely to do many of the things that can bring joy and fun to life. For those suffering from seizures, it is essential to have a high self-esteem to counter the frustration that can accompany a chronic, unpredictable health condition.

For many years, I suffered from low self-esteem. I felt inadequate when I couldn't drive. I absolutely hated to ask for a ride; I was embarrassed to take the bus, and having my mother take me to work was embarrassing as an adult. What I couldn't realize was that did not lower my value as a person. It reduced how I saw myself, it placed some limitations on what I believed I could achieve, but it had absolutely no effect on my value as an individual. It was not until I read the book "How to Be, Do, and Have Anything" by David Schwartz that I realized that I could drastically change how I felt and who I had let myself become. I realized the possibility of healing from epilepsy was there but I need to be persistent in my own holistic healing. One visit to a chiropractor or an acupuncturist was not going to heal me. Realizing that I could restore my health to what it was prior to having seizures was a huge accomplishment for me. Embracing the possibility improved my self-esteem.

> *The best day of your life is the one on which you decide*
> *your life is your own. No apologies or excuses.*
> *No one to lean on, rely on, or blame. The gift is yours –*
> *it is an amazing journey – and you alone are responsible*
> *for the quality of it. This is the day your life really begins.*
> – Bob Moawad

Increasing you self-esteem will help you enjoy your life more. Period. It can help you find ways to control your seizures better, and it will aid in making your life more employable. You will feel more confident should you need to ask for an accommodation in work, transportation, or just areas of life.

Taking responsibility for your life is a huge step in self-improvement, but it can be difficult to take that control at first. For me, I was diagnosed with epilepsy in my teenage years, so my doctors and parents dictated what I could and couldn't do in terms of activity. I was sentenced by my doctor to be on medication for the rest of my life. My self-esteem took many hits as the years went by – doling out money for medications that kept me drowsy, less effective at work, and, of course, broke. When I began to realize that I could change everything, my attitude towards life began to improve and my self-esteem began to grow.

To start to improve that self-esteem, you need to own your reality. Your health, your job, your finances, your relationships are all where they are because of YOU. It is okay to want to be somewhere different in your life, but to improve, you need to be honest with where you are right now. Recognize that the actions you took led you to this point and have created the lifestyle that you have today. You now know that you can change. You are reading this book because you know you can change.

To build up that self-esteem, you must have positive self-talk coupled with action. Let's read that phrase again. Positive self-talk coupled with action. You have adopted an abundance mentality, now you are acting on it. By becoming conscious of the messages that are going through your head, you can analyze whether they are positive or negative. You want to increase the positivity in your life and decrease the negative messages about yourself.

A great exercise for this is to create what I call a Gratitude Journal. It can be a beautifully bound, leather covered heirloom, or it can simply be a file on your computer. This Gratitude Journal will help you tune in and recall the good things you have going on in your life right now. Your mind will begin to shift and identifying positives in your life will become easier and easier. You will begin to see changes in how you view yourself after about 90 days of keeping the journal.

Additionally, create an Accomplishment Board. This is like a vision board. Write down every accomplishment, large and small, that you achieved in the last twelve months. Reflect or meditate on the list and observe how your worries fade. An Accomplishment Board builds up your confidence by being that reminder of what you have done that has value. There are simply days when you feel washed out. Powerless. You may be recovering from a seizure. In any instance, you feel wiped out and like you can't do anything. The Accomplishment Board can stand as a testimonial to you about the things you have done.

It starts simply by asking yourself, at the end of the day, "What are 3 things that I appreciate about myself?" Write down your answers every evening. Don't write the same thing each night. If you absolutely must, then expand on the idea from the night before. Reading through these things after a few weeks will give you a deeper insight into your nature and that will help to fuel this boost in your self-esteem. This goes back to the Neurowisdom ideas of Mark Waldman. Focusing on the positive things, the things that we are grateful for, for as little as twelve minutes a day, begins to change our brain chemistry and we see and feel that gratitude begin to displace the negatives. Our glass ceases to be half empty or half full, we have a new glass that runs over with abundance. We now find it easy to share that abundance because of that Abundance Mentality we have embraced. We give it away. See how this all works? We are creating a loop of positive reinforcement in our lives. As it gains momentum, we gain momentum. It is not a symptom of a positive, benevolent universe smiling back at us, but the validation of us seeking to help ourselves and others.

Using positive language in reference to yourself can often be harder since negatives tend to be programmed into us. We have a dialogue going on in our head throughout the day, and a lot of that content is to warn us of things that could happen; shifting this to a positive will bring you so much more success in life, but you have to teach yourself to do it. Usually negative thinking created fear and this fear leads to inaction. Positive thoughts and thought patterns bring progress and action. This action begets a positive cycle that you build on for life. Sometimes simply hearing positive thoughts can help you begin this process. Positive affirmations during the day can help change your habits. Thinkrightnow.com has a line of CDs to help reprogram your thinking and improve your self-confidence. You can also create your own positive affirmations, record yourself saying them and listen to them throughout the day.

Don't be afraid to try something new. You challenge yourself in a bigger way when you get outside your comfort zone. When you try something new, you may not initially be great at it, but at least you didn't stay home doing nothing. Trying new things is a great way to come alive and get out of a rut. You will appreciate yourself all the more for just trying. That can raise your self-esteem. Make it a point to regularly get outside your comfort zone. Don't go in with any expectations, just tell yourself that you will try something out.

Begin to believe in yourself. Henry Ford once said, "Whether you think you can, or you think you can't – you're right." This is one of the main reasons that it can be so detrimental to get Social Security Disability Income (SSDI). To get this disability income, you have to prove to the government that you are somehow unable to work. In doing so, you may just as easily prove to yourself that you can't work. If you don't think you can work, you probably will not even try. Cultivate the belief that you can. Create the reality that you have value.

Returning to that Gratitude Journal for a moment, use it to start proving your ability to work. Start by listing all of your skills and abilities on a sheet of paper. You may not be able to list many right then. Come back to it, add to it, study it, revise it. Write down all the things you are good at whether you are paid for them or not. You will find that you have skills that other people would pay to learn. You have knowledge other people want. You can provide a service that someone else needs. You can start making money off what you know now, and when you do, you will again feel more empowered. As you continue to listen to positive affirmations and messages on a daily basis, these will help to trigger your belief in these messages and you will seek out the habits that make these messages true from the start.

Create a positive playlist. Music can have a great impact on your attitude. There are positive, upbeat songs that will have you jumping for joy and believing in yourself. You may want to exercise to some of these songs. Get them in your head and believe in the message. When I was in elementary school, my gym teacher played Eye of the Tiger by Survivor; to this day, I still get excited when I hear it. If you enjoy the tune and it has a positive message, listening to it will have a positive effect on your self-esteem. There is a likely song for every emotion out there that can be felt. It may be a quick pick-me-up or even set the tone for a great day during a morning workout or when getting ready for work.

Start a creative project such as a piece of artwork or learning an instrument. As a person puts his heart and soul into an art project – and spends hours working on it, cultivating it, and making it beautiful – they will feel an enormous sense of accomplishment when it is complete. Those feelings of accomplishment go a long way in raising self-esteem and keeping you out of depression when a seizure does hit. In this same vein, restoration of antiques such as furniture, tools, even firearms or vehicles, can provide this same feeling, and provide a nice alternate income stream for a hobby.

All of these things require action. You simply cannot plan your way to a goal being achieved. Start to take action, even if it is a small step. This will help you eliminate the fear, increase your self-esteem, and propel you towards your goals faster. I planned this book for a long time, but I had to just sit down in front of the computer and start to write to get the actual book written. By taking action, I could eliminate the fear. Maybe the book is a best seller, maybe it is not, but I won't know until I write it. As my fear faded, my self-esteem soared. Inaction would have left me right where I was.

In all this, you must start appreciating other people and stop comparing your life to theirs. They are not you, you are not them. When you compare lives to someone without epilepsy, you start to fall into a destructive habit. You can never win in a comparison, so don't try. Someone will always be better and someone will always be worse. With that Abundance Mentality, we know there is plenty to go around! Celebrate your progress. Celebrate the action that you are taking towards your goal. Look at how far you have come instead of how far you need to go. Compare you to you! Yourself and your results. Rejoice when you have improved your results but don't lose hope because of a setback. In this way, you can continue to drive your motivation and boost your self-esteem.

Never forget to give out a compliment, and do it as often as you can. This helps you identify the wonderful things in other people and allows you to see them in yourself. You will quickly notice how the favor gets returned. People will be complimenting you on your good qualities and that, in turn, will help you realize that you have a lot to offer the world. It will help your brain focus more on the positive in your life.

That idea ties to my next one – find the upside in events, the positive in everything. We look at having a seizure and losing our license in a negative sense. While it certainly is inconvenient to have to ask other for rides, it does give them the chance to serve us. They get the positive vibe of helping another whom they may feel is not as fortunate as they are. Riding in the car with them gives them the chance to know us better. It can be an opportunity to employ a taxi driver and help him earn a living. Losing your license may force you to walk to more places. That is better for your health and better for the environment. Start turning the negatives in your life into positives. You will see that you have a wonderful life and watch your self-esteem grow.

In all these things, there is a certain amount of housekeeping in your life. All the self-esteem in the world will do you no good if you are just a liar and a cheat. Make sure you are a trustworthy person. People like to spend time and do business with those they know, like, and trust. Make sure your integrity and honesty is second to none. If you offer to pay for gas or buy lunch, do it. To this I can add to always do your best. When you are trying your hardest, you simply cannot worry about what others think of you. You need not worry about your weaknesses nor apologize for them. Never quit improving. You cannot rest on your laurels. You must continue to build on your knowledge and skills to improve your marketability in the workplace, but also to help others to see that it can be done, no matter what. Be honest, be humble, be engaged in friendship and work. I'm not telling you to be honest and engaged because you have epilepsy, I am telling you to be honest and engaged because it is the right thing to do, and as you go forward, the value you create in yourself is just another part of becoming the best individual you can be. This raises your self-esteem and creates an even more powerful belief structure, which is very important as you take the steps to heal yourself.

Spending time increasing your own self-esteem will help you feel more empowered. A higher self-esteem helps you to move outside of your comfort zone. You will begin to start accomplishing more things and trying more things. That includes making a productive contribution to society and earning a living. Having a high self-esteem enables you to enjoy life more and take better care of yourself. That healthier outlook leads to better seizure control.

*Our deepest fear is not that we are inadequate.
Our deepest fear is that we are powerful beyond measure.
It is our light, not our darkness that most frightens us.
We ask ourselves, Who am I to be brilliant, gorgeous,
talented, fabulous? Actually, who are you not to be?
You are a child of God. Your playing small does not serve
the world. There is nothing enlightened about shrinking so
that other people won't feel insecure around you.
We are all meant to shine, as children do. We were born
to make manifest the glory of God that is within us.
It is not just in some of us; it is in everyone. And as we
let our own light shine, we unconsciously give other
people permission to do the same. As we are liberated from
our own fear, our presence automatically liberates others.*
–Marianne Williamson

Habits to Stop NOW

Self-pity gets you nowhere. One must have the adventurous daring to accept oneself as a bundle of possibilities and undertake the most interesting game in the world making the most of one's best.
–Harry Emerson Fosdick

There are some things that people with epilepsy or any chronic illness must stop doing in order to elevate their lives, have successful careers, and gain enjoyment from living. They must stop the self-pity. I see lots of people posting "epilepsy sucks" in online support groups. Well, no kidding! No one signed up for it, nobody wanted it, but you have it, so deal with it. I read all the time online how awful it is to have epilepsy. Other people, people who want to help you, get tired of hearing how bad you have it. The negativity gets you nowhere. In fact, it is actually keeping you from seeing the positive and thinking about all the possibilities. Stop using negative language like "fighting" and "sucks" when you are talking about the health condition you live with. It doesn't deserve that much mental attention. Minimize how much you think about the negative aspects of it.

In his book, The Magic of Thinking Big, author David J. Schwartz recommends that we stop talking about our health problems altogether. Unless you are lifting someone up and letting them know about a positive solution, don't make comments regarding your health concerns. It is simply a waste of mental energy. Use that energy to focus on a positive solution and having gratitude for what you have and what you can do. You will find that there is more to enjoy about your life than you ever imagined.

A friend of mine told me a story about his father, who many years ago had been a coal miner in West Virginia. His dad had developed diabetes after retiring, and later, lost both of his legs due to the disease. When the son, who lived on the other side of the United States, had gone home to visit his father, he was amazed how positive his dad was about his life, even though he was in a wheelchair. He joked about how tall his sons were, he was not afraid to discuss his issues, and he embraced his "new" life. As my friend put it, "If my Dad was okay with not having any legs, I figured I had better be fine with it, too." Positive mental attitude is one of the easiest ways to change your life for the better. You need to embrace it and get on with living.

Stop going to support groups that don't offer much value. Many support groups just really are not that supportive. The next time you visit, pay attention to how much time is spent in positive conversations. If most of the people there are just complaining about the side effects and their doctors, it may be an ineffective use of your time. While it is helpful to connect with people who have experienced the same things that you have and share in your health concerns, it is far more important to your own health and well-being to stay positive. There is a tendency in some groups to start complaining about the seizures you have experienced because you have someone there who can relate. Don't get stuck in this cycle! You want to find positive solutions to your problems. Complaining about them is a waste of time. It may make you feel better temporarily as you are connecting with this new person, but it is something that keeps you trapped mentally. Spending your non-seizing time complaining about seizures gives epilepsy a greater role in your life.

I was discussing this support group criticism with a friend of mine who is a recovering alcoholic, and he started laughing! I looked at him like he was crazy and he explained. "When I first started going to AA (Alcoholics Anonymous) meetings back in 2004, I had the same problem. I didn't want to go to a group online, so I tried the ones that met in my area. The first two meetings I attended, I hated. The first group was filled with what I considered to be people that had a chip on their shoulder since I was trying to quit booze and they had quit. The next group was so intent on complaining about the first group that I got nothing even feeling like support. Finally, I found a small group close to my home that looked and sounded like me. The members had struggles, they had relapses, they had families. They became the reason that I was able to stay sober. I could relate to what they went through and I could talk to them about my troubles. It was the best part of getting sober for the first year." These are the things that make any support group work and if you aren't getting it from yours, find the one that you can actually get some value from.

Stop the habit of relying solely on your medical professional to control your seizures. Your health is so much more than taking a medication. You alone are responsible for your health. You are the one who deals with your health choices, not your doctor. Your doctor does not deal with your side effects, you do. Many natural things can be done to improve your health, and as a result increase your seizure control. We are all limited in our knowledge, and this is true of doctors as well. They are limited to how much they may know about each medication. A doctor cannot tell you how much exercise you need or how to exercise. That exercise can be a huge part of seizure control. Proper nutrition isn't in a neurologist's coursework, either, but ensuring that you have the right amount of B vitamins can lead to better seizure control. You owe it to yourself to learn all you can. Think of your health as you would think of owning a car or a house. In that ownership, you are responsible for the maintenance of it. You may not change the oil in your car, but you are responsible to get it done. Servicing the furnace in your house may be beyond the scope of your personal knowledge, but you need to know at what intervals to have it done.

You simply must learn all that you can about how to improve your overall health. That will go a long way in improving your quality of life. As your overall health improves, your productivity improves, and that is not just at work. You will be ready when the time comes to act on an invitation, you will not spend hours having to clean the house, you will be available when the boss calls for help or a client calls for a new sale. Clear thinking due to better health will lead to a myriad of opportunities and that extends to multiple sources of income and joy. Being able to recognize these chances you receive requires training yourself to recognize them.

Stop viewing your seizures as failures. Start seeing them as a reminder to improve your overall health. It is your body's way of getting rid of excess electrical activity in your brain. Don't get frustrated and start to feel like your medication isn't working and your doctor doesn't know what to do. After you visit your doctor and make a change in medication, find a healthy habit to adopt that will eliminate the toxins from your body. This could be as basic as beginning to exercise every day, ensuring that you are hydrated with proper water intake (the so-called Water Cure), and eating plenty of vegetables every day. Just taking a few positive steps on your own helps you to feel more in control over your health. It gives you peace of mind. It improves the functioning of your brain and you can focus more on solutions to everyday life.

Stop making your health an excuse to living. Quit looking at the reasons that epilepsy can somehow limit you. It will only limit you if you allow it. After failing at a job and being fired when I had done my best, I went online to see if there could be a reason that epilepsy had somehow changed my brain so it did not work "properly". In reading medical journals, I discovered that my seizures could have an impact on my memory. I also found other journals that said it was not affected. Online, I realized that I could find validation for any theory that I wanted to pursue. If you want to believe that epilepsy will negatively impact your memory and hold you back, you can find that theory somewhere. You can also find people who have overcome it naturally and completely turned their health around. You will discover people who are living full, exciting lives in spite of epilepsy and the medication's side effects.

"Bad" health is often used as an excuse when one fails to do what they want to do. You need to be mature enough to ask yourself the question, "Is epilepsy contributing to my (job, relationship, health) problem, or is that problem caused by me just not addressing it like a grown up?" I cannot run a four minute mile, but that is not because of my epilepsy. Blaming epilepsy for something that it did not contribute to is a stupid excuse, period. Be real with yourself. If you are just a bad person, then being a bad person with epilepsy is all you are. Epilepsy is a neurological disorder, not an excuse to act a certain way. If anything, you have the responsibility, wanted or not, to be better than the "regular" people who do not have to deal with a seizure event. Think of the many people who have been highly successful and have not allowed their medical condition to define them or get in their way. Danny Glover rarely talks about his epilepsy. He focuses instead on his acting career and his television and film productions. Pop icon Prince, or whatever he is being called these days, has suffered from epilepsy since childhood. He has written hundreds of songs, produced ten platinum albums, and thirty Top 40 singles in his career spanning four decades. He created a unique style of music that was rock, blues, and urban and built a niche for amazing success. The fastest woman in the world, Florence Griffith Joyner –"FloJo"- set records in the 100 and 200 meter sprints in the Olympics in 1988 that have, to this day, never been equaled or even seriously contended… but she had epilepsy. It obviously did not slow her down! You have the potential to become great and epilepsy cannot be the excuse that holds you back.

Open Your Heart

You can have everything in life you want, if you will just help enough other people get what they want.
–Zig Ziglar

Open up your heart to other people, ideas, and concepts. Start helping other people in their quest to achieve what they want even if you can only help them a little. It may sound counterproductive to start helping other people get what they want instead of focusing on what you want, but it the way to build trust. People do business with those that they know, like, and trust. It won't matter that you have a disability when someone else see that you care about them and choose to help them.

Some people with epilepsy struggle with the simple act of friendship. These people feel that friendship is always a 50-50 split, and they somehow feel they do not bring enough to the equation, so they quit trying. Asking for a ride is somehow a burden. Yes, it can be frustrating when family and friends do not understand the very real struggle we feel about transportation, but it need not define a friendship, nor is it a condition of friendship. Let that feeling of inadequacy go. I have lots of friends, some are close, so not so close. Some I can tell anything to, and some require a degree of reserve regarding a topic. I have had to let silly feelings that equate friendships into a cost-benefit analysis go. Remember what we said about scarcity? It cannot apply to friendships.

Open yourself up to other people. Learn more about them and show them that you care about them. Start reaching out to five people in your network each day. Find out how they are doing through a phone call or email. You will be surprised how quickly such a favor is returned. Suddenly, you will be receiving as you are giving. Don't be surprised if social or business invitations become a regular part of your day due to a "just thinking about you" call.

People want to see you succeed. They want to help you. The first step starts with you, though. Open yourself up. I know, I know. "I might get hurt." Yep. You might. Your feelings are not protected. You are putting them out there, and you may meet some people that just suck. If you aren't out there meeting people, it is likely that you are dwelling on a past hurt. Let it go, embrace your new self-esteem, embrace the abundances in your life, and reprogram yourself to spend time building relationships and socializing with people you like and that like you.

> *In order to have friends, you must first be one.*
> **–Elbert Hubbard**

Let's face it, people with epilepsy need friends. It can be very frustrating to try to be a friend when you are limited by walking or public transportation. You may get invited to the party, but you can't get to the party. It is just plain uncomfortable to ask for rides to an event that you would like to attend. Making those friendships seems harder when you are suffering from seizures. People are more understanding than you think. Don't take it personally when someone cannot give you a ride when you ask. They have other things going on in their lives as well. A friend of mine is a great example of how to make this work. As a teenager, he was nearly killed in a car wreck, and as a result, he has made the decision not to drive. Does it slow him down socially? Not a bit. He is a full time student, living off campus, and also has a full time job in a local restaurant. He plans his rides out a week in advance based on his schedule from school and work. He uses a large group of friends and supporters, and keeps his managers abreast of any ride situations. His employer has even helped him with rides since he has become a valuable asset for the company. By communicating with friends, employers, and professors in advance, he has built goodwill by showing that he will not use transportation as an excuse, and he doesn't.

Selfishly, being a good friend can also help you to raise awareness and of understanding of epilepsy in your circle of influence. Friends will share your story with other people if you let them know it. More importantly, you are showing them that you are not carrying the plague, you just have a little more electricity in your brain than they do, and if you get a short circuit, you need to take a break for a few minutes. People think nothing of their friends who have, say, diabetes, because we as a collective group of people know that it is a fairly common health issue that can be remedied with regular injections of insulin or just monitored carefully through diet. When you say "epilepsy", that same group of people freak out, thinking that they are going to have to do CPR in the next five minutes. By talking about it and educating others, you also educate yourself. You become more comfortable with what you can do, who you are, and in some ways, you begin to create a new you by living the standard you discuss. Thus your network of friends helps to positively reinforce this new standard of an empowered individual who has a great outlook and has an itty-bitty little seizure disorder. This network of friends now becomes a network of believers. You have shown them through your actions that you are a great person and responsible friend. Thus having that great network of friends can lead to more employment opportunities. People will tell managers about their friends who are looking for a job. People want to work with other people they like, and they hear from managers or owners first when an opening is coming up. Of course, activities with friends will also divert your attention from a seizure event or medical issues to things that are positive and have real value.

Focusing daily on opening up your heart to other people will help you become a good friend. People who know you care about them will start to care about you and your health. During my time as a substitute teacher, I often helped out at the library. I shared my book concept with the librarians. I was truly touched when the librarian told me that he had heard about new medications that could possibly help my health condition. Although I had been reluctant to share with him my weird health condition (Alopecia), I was impressed that a few months later when he heard about a new drug, he would take the time to tell me about it. When I was a member of the Fairfax Business Networking International (BNI) group, one of the members referred me to a holistic neurologist. I never would have stumbled upon her had I not been willing to share my story with the group. I truly appreciated that there was someone who cared enough to refer me to a person whose health practice was more expansive than medication alone and who specialized in epilepsy.

Many people who have a chronic illness, such as epilepsy, tend to feel dependent on others. When they can't drive, they are reliant on others to take them to medical appointments, work, and social activities. They are forced to depend on medical professionals and rely on their opinions. They often strive for independence since there is so much dependence in their lives. There is not the first thing wrong with independence. A better quality, though, is interdependence.

What is that? Interdependence, our old friend Google tells us, "is the degree to which members of a group are mutually dependent on the others in the group. Participants may be emotionally, economically, ecologically, or morally reliant on and responsible to each other." Mahatma Ghandi explains it well, "Interdependence is and ought to be as much the ideal of man as self-sufficiency. Man is a social being."

Interdependence can lead you to places that you never dreamed about. It allows you to entertain ideas that never would have occurred to you in isolation. This new interdependence can enable you to help more people and, as a result, boost your self-esteem and positivity in your life. So what are some ways that you can open up your heart and begin practicing interdependence?

It has to start by first understanding what you can offer people. You must look past your perceived limitations and think of all the things you do well. Identify things that people have told you that you do well. Do not limit yourself by just thinking in terms of an employment skill, but life skills. Do you make wonderful cakes? Helping out a friend planning a child's birthday by baking a cake not only is a nice gesture, but can be a "cash-free" payment for someone who can take you to the grocery store for the rest of your groceries for the week.

Learn how to network. "Your net worth is your network." You might feel like you can't do much to help people, but when you start meeting people at networking events, you start to hear who is good at something and what they need in order to succeed. Connecting business people with their ideal clients can help build your value. It is a skill that takes some time to cultivate, but it can help you to succeed. If you don't currently have a job, it is also a skill that will enable you to find the right one.

Keep in touch with the people that have helped you throughout your life. It is easy to shut out the world when you aren't feeling well; however, connecting with five people each day will improve your relationships and help to become a better friend and individual. It will also quietly help those "soft" or "people" skills that you are developing, too. You will start to see how much other people care about you and gain a greater perspective on life because you will be opening up and exposing yourself to other people's ideas.

Share your personal stories – they are what makes you interesting and memorable. Sharing your experiences will help others open up to you. Your story is powerful, and don't be shy about the funny things that happened, either. Nick Vujicic is a quadriplegic whose inspirational conversations are as self-deprecating as they are inspiring. Real people have odd things that happen, and even though you may have a particular story driven by epilepsy, someone may have a similar story driven by a completely unrelated issue. I didn't talk a lot about my seizures when I was a teenager. When I published my book about being seizure free naturally, I found out that a family friend that had attended my church also suffered seizures. She did not share her story because she didn't know anyone who would understand. Sharing my story in a book format has helped me to expand other people's ideas about ways to become seizure free. It has helped others to realize that a seizure disorder can impact multiple areas of your life, but it can be overcome and become a positive thing.

This book is obviously driven in large part by my personal story. I have walked this walk. I don't tell it to brag, I tell it to help other people realize that the fairy tale is real. I have condensed into these pages a life spent looking for answers that my doctor's couldn't provide me with. Along the way, there were moments of brilliance, of course. I am, after all, me. But the bigger picture is that you do not have to be a "victim" of epilepsy. You made a choice already, you decided to buy and read this book. Perhaps you will realize that all the roadblocks you see in your life are not catastrophic; they just call for a minor change; of venue, or support, or some other aspect in life and with that mental tune-up, you begin to see alternatives that you can embrace and use for the better.

We spend a lot of time talking but oftentimes not much listening. Only when we realize that communication is a two way street with one person clearly talking and one person clearly listening. You cannot listen if you are talking, writing, exercising, or checking email. Practice empathetic listening. Put yourself in another person's shoes, and listen with the goal of learning something. At the same time, gain perspective on what you are really dealing with, and express how it is such a minor part of the bigger picture of your life. They may not really have any idea of what you have gone through to get here, and you may not know what forces built them. If you are not listening, you may miss out on many wonderful strengths and trials that another person has gone through. They have a story and it is one that you should seek out. If you do not or cannot listen, you miss things that could bring you a new friend, a potential customer, or an inspirational story. It could be that they have beat a chronic disorder or a "disability." They may have been places you want to be or been places you have been. You will never know until you open your heart, take the cotton out of your ears, and put it in your mouth.

Create Your Own Support Team

Teamwork is so important that it is virtually impossible for you to reach the heights of your capabilities or make the money that you want without becoming very good at it.
–Brian Tracy, motivational speaker

The most successful people in business have mastermind groups. If you want to become successful in eliminating your epilepsy, creating a wonderful life, and excelling at employment, finding and building a team that can keep you going is very helpful. Who is on the team? We have already discussed some of them. Friends that are really friends, other people that suffer seizures, doctors, nutritionists, exercise therapists, and, like it or not, family.

Not all of our loved ones are helpful. Parents and family members are some of the most caring people. They are well-meaning, but that doesn't always mean they are supportive. Sometimes they may feel that your epilepsy is somehow their cross to bear. They will try to influence you on treatment decisions and employment opportunities based on how they think they would handle epilepsy. They can be overly critical about our choices based on their own experiences. This does not mean they are giving you bad feedback, but you must filter it. Relate to them things such as how often you have had a seizure event and how long the recovery was. Have you ever really described what a seizure felt like? Can you describe it to yourself? Thinking about this most basic part of the disorder and trying to learn how to accurately describe it can be very eye-opening to those who care about you. Think about trying to describe flight to someone who has never flown, or colors to someone who cannot see? Get the challenge of describing a seizure to someone that has never had one? Spend some time letting them know what you have … tonic-clonic, myoclonic, absence, or atonic. Educate them on what that really means. We have gotten past petit mal and grand mal, so spend some time letting those on your team know what "Epileptic" really means. This will allow them to provide better support and encouragement for you to achieve your goals.

When I started my first business in medical billing, I joined networking groups such as Business Networking International (BNI). I learned not only how networking can benefit you in your professional goals by referring business, but I made some great connections that have stayed with me. I had found another group that shared successes and struggles, but with the end goal of business growth. People listened non-judgmentally and offered words of encouragement as well as advice. It was incredibly helpful. The group met on a regular basis and all the members quickly became friends.

Creating a team to support you in your journey to heal from epilepsy, gain meaningful employment, and achieve your personal and professional goals is a process. You may not find very much support in an epilepsy support group, especially if the conversation wallows in self-pity, complaining about medications and side effects, and is really just a bunch of whiners. We all know that the anticonvulsants cost a lot, have side effects, and any change in a prescription can bring on a whole host of new issues. Do not be afraid to create a support group that is not really even a formal group. It may only be a social group that meets for coffee, or a small cadre of people from a local church. It does not need to have a title. It may only be the circle of caring individuals that rarely meet as a group. What is important is that they all gain from you and that you derive a feeling of empowerment from their positivity.

Decide what you want to accomplish with this team. Do you want support getting off medication and controlling seizures naturally? Find or build your local group on natural healing and start making friends there. Are you searching for a home based income solution? Get to know people in that field through networking groups online or in person. When you feel like you have encountered someone that has knowledge of things in alignment with your goals, invite them for a coffee. If they are not local, Skype them and have a virtual cup of coffee. Make sure you stay in touch with them. Call, text, or email at least once a week. Find out what they may need help with and offer support wherever and however you can. We all know that patients with complex medical issues have entire teams of doctors working together for their health and treatment, I am telling you to do the same thing, but with people that help you in achieving your goals. Not only should your doctors be on your team, but also, natural healers and, even more importantly, friends and business contacts.

This broad network of individuals that are helping you should also have the benefit of you passing them referrals in business or life. You may have a friend undergoing treatment for cancer, so you should introduce them to a cancer survivor you know. That cost nothing, but the hope you may have given someone is priceless; on the other hand, you may have someone in your network looking for a new home, and you can introduce them to a realtor that you know and trust, and that may result in a small finder's fee if the realtor sells to your referral. At any rate, this team should be people you feel good about and one that keeps you positive because they are positive. You should feel comfortable around them and be able to share aspects of your life that you do not discuss with the naysayers that are all around. It should include people that coach you, that you can coach, and people offering positive influences and alliances.

In all this I team building I sought out people and things that could prevent seizures. I researched what I knew about my own body, then sought out the expertise of acupuncturists, chiropractors, naturopaths, and other alternative healers to share their wisdom with me and expand my knowledge. They supported my goal of coming off medication. They rejoiced in my triumphs and helped me get back on track when things did not go as I thought they should. I got healthier and healthier because I had people who had different expertise that I lacked and making suggestions that I never would have come up with on my own. I did not rely only on what I knew, I found trustworthy people that could actively help me pursue my goal of better overall health and I found trustworthy friends that actively encouraged that new lifestyle.

Be willing to invest in that team. BNI does have a nominal cost associated with membership. Hiring a chiropractor and a nutritionist costs money. However, that money I spent in order to receive expertise and participate in the networking group was inconsequential compared to the amount of value that I received from the group. I often hear of people who aren't willing to try an alternative healing method because it isn't covered by their health insurance. They are only limiting themselves. The cure that they are so desperately looking for may be found with a few trips to an acupuncturist. Sometimes a chiropractor may mention something that you go home and research and decide to implement in your life. It makes you feel better, and you become more productive and happier. I would say that it is probably worth the cost of the visit!

*Teamwork is the secret that makes
common people achieve uncommon results*
–Ifeanyi Enoch Onuoha, Infopreneur and coach

Many people who have epilepsy think that I am full of something not socially acceptable to discuss when I tell them I am seizure free and medication free. They tell me that not everyone can do it. With the right team in place, you can accomplish anything. It does take persistence. In the process, you will make great friends, expand your mind, and improve your health. Your team members will celebrate your victory. Even though some of the people on my team were paid professionals, that still did not stop me from taking them out to dinner outside of our working relationship. Knowing how much an attorney I had used loved breakfast pastries, if I was near his office in the morning, it was not unusual for me to drop off a cheese danish for him. Did I do it every day? Of course not. I might do it once every two or three months. It was the thought that counted, and that is the idea I am conveying here. Remember your team. You are the one building it, put the players on it you need.

Start a networking group for one of your own interests or hobbies. Find a restaurant to meet at and make sure that you remember they are there to make money, so be sure to make it worth the business' time to have you. Many restaurants that open for lunch have staff in them as early as 7 or 8 a.m., so ask the owner or manager if you could use their dining room for a meeting and have a server come in to handle coffee. Let them know you will pay for the products you use and take care of a gratuity for the wait staff. Think of and share tips on the interests you and the rest of the group share. When people begin to show and join, make them feel welcome and embrace their skills. It need not have a thing to do with epilepsy.

That can be a footnote on what you share about that hobby. The other members will appreciate it and will help to support you in other endeavors that you are involved in. If you don't think you are an expert at something, Google it! Use your local resources at the library or online and figure it out. Your team members will celebrate your victory and respect you all the more for it. Share what you have learned about whatever topic you are the expert on, and see what others think about it. This helps to add to the feeling of empowerment and the abundance mentality we discussed earlier. As an added bonus, since you selected the location, transportation is not an issue and you have built more fans at that business.

Build Your Offensive Line

Still with me? Great! Because we have covered a lot of ground, but a lot of it is in your head. Getting your mind right is a huge part of this game. At some point, though, you have to DO something. A job, a family, a life. We are going to explore a lot of the job and employment options in the last parts of the book, but it makes no sense to talk about how employable you are and give you ideas for managing a job if you don't have your mindset right for the rest of the hours in your week. I had to get you in the abundance mentality, make you build your self-esteem, get you some good habits and some new ideas to try. Now is the first of the serious stuff. You have built that support team of doctors, friends, family, maybe even a networking group that doesn't rely on your seizure disorder for content to talk about. You need to have some long talks with three very important people. Your attorney. Your accountant. Your insurance agent. I call them the Offensive Line because, like their namesake on the football field whose only job is to protect the quarterback, their only job is to protect you, the client.

These three folks are the key to maintaining something of value that you built in your life. It doesn't matter if you have $500 or $500,000 to pass along, you need to look at all your legal and financial strategies to keep more of what you make. One key thing to remember is that you get what you pay for in these fields. Hire the best you can afford. I think of them in the sense as an umbrella or a fire extinguisher. When you really need one, nothing else will do.

Where do you start? I would go locate an attorney in your state and engage him or her for an hour to discuss who you are, what you do for a living, where you are financially, where you are going financially, and what protections you may or may not need. This may sound strange, but find an attorney who is around your age. This will lead to common life events (marriage, children, grandchildren, etc…) and it will help to ensure that they "speak your language". It will do you no good to sit down to build a long term relationship with a legal expert who will be retiring in five years, additionally, by getting the "younger" specialist, you are getting somebody that may not be locked into old theories and ideas that are outdated. You are not putting this firm on retainer, you are seeking their advice and crafting a long term strategy for legal protections. You may use them for a will, incorporating a company (which we will cover later), and other legal needs that someone would reasonably need. Don't forget that part of this meeting is about setting specific goals for your life. If you will be building or buying a business in the next year, get ahead of the curve by having that discussion. I strongly recommend that you sit down with "your" attorney at least once a year on the state of your life. They can advise you on things that you may need to consider before you hit certain milestones – legal protections about age begin at 40, for example.

Of course, you may not be at a place where you need to do that right this second. Perhaps you are still in school, perhaps you are just embarking on a career or have not built a gameplan. A great resource then may be a company like LegalShield, which I have included in the resources section. They can help start the process of legal and identity theft protection without getting tied down to a particular firm yet.

The next person on the Offensive Line is your accountant. The same rules of age and experience apply here. You want one that you can grow old with. They are great for the basics of a tax return with a plain Form 1040 for a W-2 employee, but they really shine when you are building your own business. In preparing for this book, I had a long talk with a young man who has just recently finished all his CPA tests and coursework, Chase Ward of Atlanta, Georgia. I was pretty blunt with him about epilepsy and the fact that so many of us have gotten some disability benefit and now are limited to only working a certain amount of hours weekly (usually 25) which pretty much guarantees that we aren't going to retire rich. I was very surprised at his responses-

"The first thing is to look at is what the individual wants to, and can legally, do. There are very specific things that can be done with and S- or a C-Corporation (two types of traditional small business incorporation), and if the individual that runs that small business corporation is careful in the disbursement of dividends from that entity; he or she can process, that is to say, use the funds from that business to write off certain deductions such as a home office, a vehicle, and a substantial amount of other aspects of, shall we say, day-to-day costs. This would, for tax purposes, be seen as company expenses, not dividends, and may be used for the betterment of the company and any benefit to the individual due to these purchases or expenditures may not be taxable. The tax code of the United States is always changing, and how so-called "unearned income" is seen can change from year to year and, sadly, from accountant to accountant. I cannot stress enough that any individual choosing to do this must be aware of the different laws in different states. As an example, the states of Wyoming and Nevada have laws very supportive of small business, while Delaware has a fantastic protections for traditional larger corporations. While I may be an expert at this from my desk, your readers must speak to their accounting firm specifically to find out details with respect to state tax laws."

In a nutshell, you can build a business, incorporate it, be successful at it, and still keep the SSDI benefits you potentially spent years to get. There are plenty of hurdles you will have to jump through, and you simply must have a relationship with an accountant that knows tax law, corporate law, and the relationships that SSDI can play in your unearned income. It is simply too complex to diagnose in one book, much less a part of a chapter. If you do not spend the time to find the right "teammates" for your offensive line, you will never know what can be done and how you can grow and protect a financial legacy for you and your family. As this was going to press, Mr. Ward was beginning the process of building a spreadsheet to be able to project income and then protect income strategies based on certain levels of SSDI against C- and S-Corporation taxation. It sounds like a bad accounting test, but these are the sorts of people that you need on your Offensive Line. They do not just sit in the status quo, they take their clients' needs very seriously and look for ways to make or save them money. Clearly Mr. Ward is one of the best.

The last of the big players you need on the line is your insurance agent. In this instance, we are discussing life insurance. How many times have we been told we can't get it? Plenty. Some companies simply won't insure you. So sit down with an agent, specifically one that is not trying to "sell" you, and learn about what they offer. Some companies have a very specific rules regarding the issuance of a life insurance policy to someone who suffers from epilepsy. Your job is to find out if that agent knows their company standard, and if you are not insurable, what firms will consider your case.

As an example, I spoke to Presley Lomax, a long time agent for a well-known firm. After checking with the underwriters, he explained that someone who averages a seizure a year can expect to be insured, assuming they are qualified through the underwriting process. Two or more seizure events would bar you from coverage with some firms, but not all. If you can qualify for a term life policy (the most basic standard policy of most insurance companies), he strongly recommended locking in what he called a long term convertible policy that would base the coverage on your condition now, not as it might be in ten or twenty years. This type of policy starts out as a term life policy, but you can convert portions of it to whole life as you desire. When you find your health improving, you can always cancel that policy as you go back through the underwriting process so they look at your current health scenario and potentially lower the premium you are paying. In a different scenario, you could convert that term policy into a whole or universal life policy as your financial situation changed or improved. He followed up with the fact that there are a multitude of firms out there who view different physical disorders with a different standard, so someone with epilepsy should seek out an expert in the life insurance field and understand what is available. The key is that you need to find an agent that is not just trying to sell you insurance. He or she should be educating you on what policies mean what. Universal? Term? Whole Life? In the case that you simply are not able to get a policy in your name, that agent should have the ability to guide you through the options available for a spouse, a child, and long-term care. Mr. Lomax's contact information is included in the Resources section in the back of the book.

In all this, remember, you are the client. You have an active role to play in this. They work for you to develop strategies to protect you and your family, to increase your wealth, to plan your estate, and to understand the very real issues you face. You owe it to yourself to become an expert on what you employ them to do. If you read about potential legal proceedings with SSDI or protections offered under ADA (Americans with Disabilities Act) or its equivalent in your state or country, for example, you should be emailing them the information and planning a follow up call with each after they have the chance to check out the material. They should each know how their advice will affect and react with the advice of the other members. Therefore, they should all be clear on the gameplan of the others and their advice must be complimentary to the entire group. Remember, you are not the smartest person in the room, but they should all be developing plans based on the common set of goals you have outlined for you, your family, and your company.

Learn about all your responsibilities as a client. Have a meeting with all of them at the table, so they can all understand the goals you have set; for your life, your job or company, and how you are building a legacy for your family. This game plan will be the foundation of your path to financial success, and should be at least an annual meeting. These three people are on your Christmas list. They may not interact with your other team very often, but these professionals are a very important group to you. Remember that.

Tapping into Your Creative Side

*Most people spend more time and energy
going around problems than trying to solve them.*
–Henry Ford

There have been many times in my life when I was mentally derailed by the thought of losing my license or caught up worrying how I could possibly get anywhere when the real answer was simply to know that all I needed to do was to phone a friend and ask for a ride, walk to my destination, or just hop on the bus. Solutions to our problems are out there if we just look for them. It just may require a bit of creativity. Tapping into our creative side regularly gives us more practice in the act of being creative. That may seem obvious, but by thinking outside the box, we begin to see opportunities and solutions that we may have ignored when we just went through life as a part of a routine. There are many jobs out there for the creative minority. You never have to be unemployed if you are willing to do one of the three things : change the work that you are offering to do, change the place you are offering to work, or change the amount that you ask for your services. In short – adapt!

If you try to do something and fail, you are vastly better off than if you had tried nothing and succeeded
–Anonymous

Aristotle, one of the most famous of the Greek philosophers and one who wrote extensively on such varied subjects a government, ethics, biology, poetry, theatre, Zoology, physics, and metaphysics suffered from epilepsy. He was the first to suggest that there is a link between epilepsy and genius, stating that they go hand in hand. According to him, the seizures that wracked his body and mind helped to activate parts of the brain that were involved in creativity. Seek out what you are good at and pursue it, don't dwell on your epilepsy, which is a mere medical condition that has not stopped a long list of people from achieving greater heights.

"But I'm just not very creative and I really can't think around corners to solve problems…" Nonsense. Creativity is a skill that can be developed, honed, and utilized. It is just like a muscle that needs to be exercised because it may have grown weak. The most creative people are usually the people who are problem solvers. These people, from all areas of life, can tap into that creative side and are usually rewarded financially for that creativity. Everyone whether they have epilepsy or not should tap into their creative side.

So this creativity can help you financially, but just as importantly, it can help you to find solutions to health problems. Sometimes just a change in diet or activity can be the answer to seizure control. Many people firmly believe that only a doctor holds the key to a health problem. Patients quietly take the advice of their doctor and live with the outcome. There are thousands of alternatives to "standard" treatments, and we have already discussed many of them. Combining different approaches may be just what your body needs to get back in balance. When you begin to think creatively, you can find the best possible solution.

In order to become more creative, you must start doing things that creative people regularly do. They create. Start with doodling. I have a friend who recognized the power of doodling in the workplace. Discovery Doodles can teach you how to tap into your creative side, unleash your mental blocks, and doodle your way to success. Doodleinstitute.com can teach you how to powerfully represent your ideas visually. Even if you think you can't draw, at least doodle a visual representation of your idea. No one has to see it. Problems that are abstract, such as relationships with someone or a heavy workload, will benefit the most from being turned into a sketch. Cartooning using exaggerated shapes and simple symbols can really help to manifest a complex issue. This can help you better grasp the concepts and share them with others. This professional level of the Doodleinstitute teaches you to make money with doodles. Apart from monetary gains and the creative aspect, doodling can be very therapeutic and can aid in dealing with emotions.

If doodling isn't your thing, make a collage. Take a stack of newspapers and look for photos and ads that have a relationship to your problem or challenge and glue them to a poster board. Keep it near your desk where you can ponder it. It may help you achieve a new perspective on your problem or goal.

Pick up a book that has ideas you have never before considered and start reading it. Exposing yourself to new and exciting ideas is one way to create new neural pathways and start thinking creatively. I remember the moment when I started to seriously consider the idea that I could heal myself naturally. I had read Kevin Trudeau's book, "Natural Cures They Don't Want You to Know About". It fueled my drive and desire to get my own body to heal itself rather than subjecting myself to medication for the rest of my life. Was there a bunch of odd things in there? You bet. The funny thing was, nothing in the book was unobtainable, so I could embrace many of the cures with day-to-day items. It acted as an inspiration to me that there were a lot of ways that I could positively impact my health that I had never thought of.

Go to a business networking event. Whether you have a business to promote or not, meeting new people is a fun and exciting way to gain new ideas. As an example, I met an ADHD Life Coach in a BNI group some years ago. I never would have thought that there was an economic side to the ADHD debate, but she had written several books and felt called to share how she had changed her life and learned to focus past the troubles of her disorder. She created her own industry, and she had a great supply of the raw materials that she needed to be successful. Many business owners in networking groups are forthcoming to the group about their searches for good employees. They know the members of the group are supportive, so rather than take out an advertisement, they ask the members is they know of people with the skills they are seeking. Simply making friends with entrepreneurs can help you catch an entrepreneurial vision. They may even be great mentors who can help guide you on a path that you never considered before. Hanging out with people who are networking will help you elevate your life and create a bigger dream for yourself. You may find that it will help pull you out of a mental rut if you are stuck. As you interact and network with successful people, you will start to adopt their habits. Using those habits you see them model, you are in a good position to become a top earner regardless of a health condition.

Take a class that will encourage you to cultivate your creativity and learn something new. I have taken pottery classes, watercolor and painting classes, Pilates, yoga, even pole dancing. Learning to create something beautiful or a health class can stimulate your mind. This will help to broaden your horizons and will aid in encouraging you to think laterally. Not only do these things increase creativity, but taking classes improves your skill set. As your skill set increases, so does your ability to earn money. After taking a class in swimming, I was able to become a swim instructor for group and private lessons. This course was only eight weeks, but it gave me an additional revenue stream that I loved doing in my spare time. I found a fun class in Pilates and that inspired me to begin teaching Pilates as well.

Stop trying to brainstorm and start moving your body. Your brain is more engaged and active when you are moving. The old business practice of brainstorming as a powerful way to generate creativity is now seen to be less useful than in years past. Instead, try new approaches to creative problem solving. Go for a walk. Physically move your body to a different location and consider different aspects of your problem. Physical movement has now been shown to have a positive effect on creative thinking. Theatre professionals often suggest practicing lines when you are in different positions to generate new character approaches. Inspiration happens when you are out doing things. When you are mowing the lawn, taking a shower, or even walking the dog. Your brain is more active and thoughts occur to you in a different way when you are doing things. The larger the variety of things you do, the more creative you can become.

A word about brainstorming. While it has generally fallen out of practice in business, a new version of it has gained some traction, and that is "Liestorming". As silly as it sounds, it is the same idea as brainstorming, but to throw out blatant lies about things, as quickly as possible, and the stranger the better. Instead of trying to think of a unique aspect of a product for a benefit, think of a variety of things that the product can most certainly NOT do. A house cannot make your complexion better. A car will not make you lose weight. A book is not purchased because it kills bugs. By thinking out into the absurd, some real truth is usually found. If you are a long-haul truckdriver, you are not going to be able to discuss the job of a Sous chef in Manhattan… but you could certainly discuss truckstops across the nation and the food served in them. Simply start at the absurd and work back to reality. It is honestly fun to do, and expect to make yourself and the people helping you do it laugh. If you aren't laughing when you do it, you aren't doing it right. A friend of mine who sells mobile homes used to do this with other salespeople to build new sales techniques for his pitch to potential buyers. If you heard them practice these pitches, you would be amazed and appalled at the creativity they had, but when the time came to close a sale, they had created some great tools.

It may sound silly, but use toys to inspire your creativity. Many design companies encourage employees to keep toys on their desks. This could be Play-doh, Legos, Lincoln Logs, or origami paper. Taking a break from typing to physically build something with your hands can give you a creative jolt that pushes you from "good" to "great". No toys? Start writing short pieces of work quickly. There are online flash fiction groups that encourage you to quickly write a piece of fiction of about 100 words. The more you write, the better you get it at it. Stephen King got eight books out of the poem "Childe Roland to the Dark Tower Came" by Robert Browning.

Whatever you do, try to generate lots of ideas quickly. If you bought this book to help you improve your physical health, quickly write a list of as many resources as you can think of now to help you with that. When we start taking about jobs and employability, make that list. You can do this list for any common object or solution or health issue. Set a timer for five minutes. Don't worry about whether the idea is good, bad, or even viable. Some ideas will be impossible, it doesn't matter. Just see what you can come up with.

Set aside time each day for doing this sort of thing. Block out about thirty minutes each day when you are relaxed, sharp, and undistracted. The author of "The Artist's Way," Julia Cameron, recommends freewriting in a journal. If you do this on a regular basis for ninety days, you will notice that you have lots of new ideas creeping into your mind. These can help you in your problem solving and idea generation.

What do you do with these ideas? Turn them into something. Create a collage, a book, a poem, or just a doodle out of your idea. It's a way of thinking through making, a process that often leads to new ideas. Creativity is a great way to help you break out of a cycle or rut that is keeping you stuck. Creativity and empowerment work together by providing alternative ways of thinking and exploring other solutions to your problem. You may discover that you have a solution that can be very profitable and help many other people who are in a similar situation to yourself. You may figure out a service that meets the needs of your friends that you can monetize. You may realize that a service you have provided to friends and family has a larger monetary side to it and can be charged for to a larger group, and those friends and family are now helping you advertise it.

Raising Your Value

By now you may have noticed that I am offering you a roadmap to rebuilding you. We started by showing you how to get your mind right, then your body, and now we are going to look at how to get your career moving in a positive direction. Your education, knowledge, skills and experience are all investments in your ability to contribute a value for which you can be paid.

The reality is that many people with a chronic illness feel defeated. They start to feel that they have no value to add to their workplace and those suffering from epilepsy are not alone in this respect. They may begin to feel they are being discriminated against and start to examine the laws for equal employment opportunity enforcement situations. These people seem to feel that a workplace environment should be tailored to their disability and this idea is perpetuated by lawyers and people in support groups.

The reality is that if an employer has to spend too much extra time or money managing and making accommodations for one employee, they could go out of business. It is a huge disservice to the economy to start suing employers when you feel that there is discrimination due to a health issue. That employer took a risk to start the business and is likely employing others. A lawsuit diverts the energy and focus of the business and takes funds away from the business which could help in hiring and training other employees.

In the course of writing and researching this book, I interviewed two Human Resource Directors of medium size businesses. One was the hospitality industry (restaurants) and one in real estate. Both stated plainly that epilepsy was not an issue to hiring, but, as with any other health condition, could be an issue with retaining employment if the employee had numerous absences. The decision to terminate employment would be reached when the basic job functions of the description could no longer be counted on to be addressed by the employee. My question for both was the same, if an employee was terminated for a medical condition and sued for wrongful termination, what would their firm do in response?

The first company stated that they would "pay to win", that is, string out the lawsuit for so long in the legal system that the former employee would have no real recourse but to settle out of court for a small sum. The former employee would essentially lose years in the fight and the only real winner might be the counselor for the employee. Additionally, the fact that most employees cannot afford great attorneys, and many attorneys do not want to fight large companies, a legal misstep and a mistrial are always a possibility, resulting in no monetary awards.

The second company actually used a binding arbitration agreement in the hiring paperwork for employees, but the result was the same. String out the process for years, wait for a legal mistake, and get a mistrial ruling or pay a relatively small fee at the end of years of litigation. In several cases, what the employee was left with after legal fees was a great deal less than what they would have earned over the course of the legal fight if they would just have gone to work.

In both cases, any decision would be coupled with a non-disclosure agreement and a gap in employment that would be difficult to explain positively.

A much better way is to increase your value in the workplace. Look for ways to make the workplace environment better and become an asset to the business. There are so many ways to do this; from educating yourself in the many different facets of the job to simply going the extra mile when performing a task. Make the most of your "good" days at work so you build some value for when you have a tough day physically.

One of the simplest things that you can do to add value to your workplace is to supersize your greeting. That means when you meet someone, greet them with a big, genuine smile. When they ask you how you are doing, use some positive superlatives. Even though you are at work, you can still be doing wonderful, fantastic, and great. I still remember the greeting I got in a little family restaurant in the deep South while traveling years ago, "I am simply marvelous, and I hope your day is half as fantastic". For some reason, that greeting has stuck with me for many years. It is always nice to hear that someone is doing well. A smile always raises the spirits of other employees around you. Being congenial at work leads to better feelings about you as an employee. This is a strategy that I began using when I was substitute teaching. Before long, I was put on the preferred substitute list without even knowing it. I got asked by many teachers to fill in for them. My "part time" job became full time very quickly. Not only did my supersized greeting brighten the day of the folks around me, but I actually started enjoying the job that I had previously felt was just boring.

The simple fact of the matter is that employers are more likely to keep someone around and be patient with them if they are a positive influence at work. Think about how we have already discussed avoiding the friend whose life is a train wreck. The workplace is no exception. Your boss is far more likely to be willing to teach you and work with you until you shine at your job when you are a positive influence, even if you experience a seizure there or miss some time due to recovery. There were two different workplaces where I had a seizure, but neither of my employers made a big deal about it. They obviously showed concern, and wanted to make sure that they had not helped to cause it through scheduling or overwork, but were always delighted to have me back. A positive attitude can melt away the discrimination that may be initially present because people like being around those who have a positive attitude.

You can also raise your value in the workplace by going the extra mile to ensure that customers and clients are happy. Make sure they are getting what they want and that little something extra. Good customer service is an essential part of a successful business. If you have an employer, they may be your customer. They are the ones paying you for your work, so make sure they are very satisfied with your performance. It is counter-productive to start demanding accommodations for a disability from an employer who really isn't satisfied with your ability to perform the job in the first place. If you do need a special workplace accommodation, make sure you are over-delivering on your performance. Work a little later, get projects done before deadlines, spend time to understand objectives. This will help to show that your employer has hired a great employee who is doing the best they can do. In this same vein, make sure you are a team player. Work well with your co-workers and be a positive influence on them. Sometimes simply being polite is enough, sometimes you need to help complete projects or follow through on issues outlined in a conversation. Jump on opportunities that you are presented with.

Step up and step in. Ask for duties that are above and beyond the scope of what you normally do. Learn about other projects within the office or business and see if you can help. If such a chance is afforded you to help, make sure your work is accurate and helpful. The more enthusiastic you are to assist others, the more valuable you become to the business. When they appraise your value, you want to be seen as a knowledgeable asset who is known for help, not hindrance.

This all starts at the interview stage of your employment. You begin to prove you are capable of doing the job by resolving all accessibility issues and concerns before then. You want to show employers that you can and do take personal responsibility to handle transportation. They cannot legally ask if you own a car, they can only ask if you have reliable transportation to and from work. This should be an easy "yes". When the subject of epilepsy and seizures comes up, you should also be able to demonstrate that you will be as independent as possible in creating the accommodations you need on the job in case of a seizure event. Be proactive in gaining and furthering the education in technology which you need to be competitive in the job. Know how to resolve or manage problems in a wide variety of settings, such as home or at work. An employer does care about your health and safety, but they did not get into business to merely become your caretaker and provide you with health insurance. Make sure you provide value to their business and you need never worry about your role in that business.

You can raise that value by continuing to learn new skills once you have mastered the ones necessary for the performance of your current job. When I was a volunteer for Adaptive Aquatics, my performance was exceptional. When the time came for the instructor to transfer, the recreation center offered the position to me and paid for my training. After a year of demonstrating excellent instruction to children with disabilities, they offered me more hours as a regular instructor and paid for my certification in first aid and lifeguarding.

At one point, I had a scary double vision/aura seizure episode at the pool, but the recreation center had been so happy with my performance that they simply made sure I was alright and never said a word about firing me or limiting my duties. They certainly asked and made sure that I could continue to do the job that I was hired to do, but they never considered terminating me. The idea of having to find another employee after investing so much time and money in training me made little sense to them, and they continued to be a great employer since they were very happy with how

I handled my responsibilities on the job. The vertigo episode had been an expected side effect of the anticonvulsant I was taking at the time, and in hindsight, it was only a minor bump in the road.

As I increased my swimming instructor skills and the recreation center invested more time in me, I started to find other opportunities that interested me as well. I discovered classes in personal training and Pilates instruction. I educated myself on how to teach Pilates and discovered many additional job openings and chances to make money.

In all this talk of raising your value, it is important to remember that you will get feedback through evaluations and "in the field" moments. Make sure if you are being counseled for performance or even terminated that you understand why that is happening. If you do not know why they are displeased with your ability to do the job, you will never know how to fix that issue. I continuously made this mistake at several jobs in my early career over and over. I was quickly fired from a secretarial position on Capitol Hill. Rather than asking what it was that I was doing wrong, I simply pleaded to get another chance because I was just figuring things out. I got two weeks of reprieve, but I still was fired because even though I was trying harder, I still had not corrected the things that my boss felt I was doing wrong.

A secondary aspect of this may also be that your boss doesn't know how to give you proper feedback. We have a tendency to see people in positions of responsibility as somehow "all-knowing", when in reality, they may be making it up as they go along. If you are receiving a reprimand, ask what the behavior was that was wrong, and make sure you ask what is the correct behavior. If you weren't trained properly, now would be a good time to ask for some training or a review of the information.

It takes strength to be able to listen to criticism and make improvements when necessary. If you are working for an employer and they tell you that you seem disengaged or you aren't taking down information correctly, make sure that you understand what you are supposed to be documenting in order to be successful. If you take their feedback and still don't improve, it may not be the right opportunity for you. It can be tough to find a new job, but each opportunity is a chance to grow and develop new skills.

The simple fact is that employers do not get rid of those employees that add value to their organization. By building your value at work, you will ensure that you have a position as long as the company exists. It puts you in demand, then it empowers you to continue to build your value.

Another rule to remember is that businesses hire those people that they like, know, and trust. They do business with other companies for the same reasons. To increase your value in the workplace, foster a growing network friends, coworkers, and associates that help to build your net value by their ties to you. Getting to know people can be done through sports activities, networking, Meetup.com, fundraisers, Facebook, and LinkedIn. Get involved and volunteer with these activities. Ask your boss if you can help coordinate of be the contact person for your company at these events. This will build the company's trust in you and allow you to and build your network as well. You can be the face of the company and that can be a great insurance policy against termination, especially if you are a solid performer in the office.

Dale Carnegie's "How to Win Friends and Influence People" can be especially helpful in getting people to like you. You should first become genuinely interested in other people. Learn to remember people's names. A person's name is the sweetest sounding and most important sound in any language. Become an excellent listener and encourage others to talk about themselves. Talk with other people about their interests. Sincerely make other people feel important.

Workplace Environments

Now, we all have different dreams for an ideal job. I love to teach and write, so that is a huge part of my ideal job. Others dream of a home business that gives them the flexibility to work no matter how they feel. Many others, for a variety of reasons, will choose a traditional workplace or office environment. We have already looked at a number of aspects of this job area in the last chapter, but what does it really mean to be a valued employee?

First, you need to determine what kind of environment you can handle. Some places just aren't good spots to have a seizure. Construction sites are a valid place to not be when that moment comes. Just as dangerous would be a position in outside sales that requires driving from one appointment to the next. We all know that driving with a seizure disorder can be likened to Russian Roulette, so jobs that require operating a vehicle or heavy equipment is not the place to start filling out applications. If your condition is controlled with medication and your seizures are infrequent, you may be able to use a vehicle in your working environment. However, you do run the risk of losing that form of income if you have a seizure and your license is suspended, so it would be wise to have a plan if that happens. If you have your mind set on these fields, look at all the people behind those jobs. The salesman in his car probably has a staff in an office to handle his leads on new clients.

The contractors at a job site certainly have a staff offsite in an office. Here your knowledge of the business is valuable and useful. Companies that hire support staff like and utilize that staff and find it especially useful if that staff understands the business in the field or the jobsite. For someone with active seizures and a desire to be in sales, you may need to consider retail, where you are in a more controlled environment should something occur. Likewise, if you are driven to work in hospitality, a job serving or greeting would be much better than cooking in the case of a seizure, which could result in severe burns. You have to consider your own health when you consider a job and the environment you will be working in. Most of us may consider a receptionist as an ideal position, but answering the phones, assigning tasks, and making appointments may be hard for some people to juggle. Depending on the type of seizures you suffer from, striking your head on a desk corner or falling on a sharp object could be a real hazard in this environment.

The next issue to contemplate is the number of the seizures you have and what brings them about. If the stress of the job is triggering your seizures, then you may have little choice but to look into jobs creating less stress. There may be a wealth of them in the very field you are already employed in, and even in the company you are already with. Love animals but struggle at a pet store? Dog walking is a service that many busy dog lovers need which really can reduce stress and reinforce a healthy lifestyle choice. You can quickly build your own client list and create your own business or you can sign up online and work with a service that helps to find you clients. Rover.com is an online resource for dog owners that helps people post and find others that offer services related to dogs and dog ownership. This includes jobs where you can pet sit overnight while pet owners are on vacation. If you are looking to reduce stress and hate dogs, this may not be a good fit for you, but the example is here to give you ideas. If you have construction skills or real estate experience, think about home inspections for buyers and sellers. These are generally a 2-4 hour inspection of the structure to check all the systems in it. With the ability to upload photographs and publish online, a very nice looking report can be generated quickly and the client has a clear understanding of the strong and weak points of the property.

Speaking of publishing, there are many outlets for people who are skilled at writing and the graphic arts. A home environment may prove much less stressful if you are capable of creating work and adhering to deadlines. There are websites to advertise your skills and bid on jobs. A very popular one is Elance.com. If you are capable of doing jobs quickly for not a lot of money, you can advertise on Fiverr.com and start building a client base there.

So far, we have really drilled down on the stress of the job or the physical environment that it is performed in. You also need to consider the environment from co-workers. You may find yourself stressing out as a response to how negative others in that workplace are behaving. You have two choices when this occurs. The first is to be the change you want to see in your co-workers and job environment. Model the behavior that you are expecting others to show and hope that people see it and begin to change for the better. Say positive things when you get to work, have positive affirmations posted in your workspace. I have a positive message flashing every second on my computer monitor so that my subconscious mind is exposed to more positive messages (You can get this type of messaging software at ThinkRightNow.com). The second way is to fire that job and find another one in the field that offers a more positive work environment. You already know who your competition is, go interview them and see if their office is more positive. You have to consider many things in a job change, and a lot of them are hard to put a value on. Feel comfortable with the places you have to work!

Your work environment should be as safe as possible if you suffer from seizures. Spend time to educate your co-workers about your disorder. You have a responsibility to them to not have them "freaking out" if you do have an episode. Let them know what it is, what to expect, and not to get too concerned unless some specific items happen. This can save disruption at the office and prevent a well-meaning employee calling an ambulance when you just needed to relax for a few minutes and recompose yourself. Make sure that they have your emergency information and don't make them more nervous about your possible seizure than you are.

Another area that is important in your environment is your boss. Just as you are training your co-workers, train the management staff on what to expect. They have time and money invested in your skills at the job, and by letting them know that you can make up missed shifts, work extra when you are not dealing with a seizure event, or simply that you are available for other areas of responsibility you can help to validate their decision to hire you or simply keep you on board. By showing that you understand that epilepsy places some burdens on your workload and bringing solutions about that issue to them, you can actively show them that you are invested in the business and the job as much or more as any other employee.

The few times I have had a seizure at work were actually "better" than being alone. I simply told the people I worked with what might happen, what they could do if it did happen, and made sure they knew how much help they were when it did actually happen. By preparing them, I was fostering good will in the office and creating an informal team of supporters that I could call on if needed. Most times, that event never came, but I had empowered them and myself to keep me working.

A Home-Based Income

Your time is precious, so don't waste it living someone else's life.
–Steve Jobs

We have spent the majority of this book becoming empowered to take control of the life we have. We are meeting our basic physiological and safety needs, we are handling our needs for belonging, but as we climb up Abraham Maslow's Hierarchy of Needs, we find that we still feel the need for Esteem and Self Actualization. In addition to that, we, as epilepsy sufferers, often need alternative solutions to traditional employment in order to generate enough income just to live on. In that conversation, we often realize that we want more out of the jobs we "can" have and with seizures making daily life difficult, we may choose to build a business at home.

A radical example of success that was from an odd direction is Susan Boyle. She had suffered from epilepsy since childhood and had been told that her problem was a mental defect. She lived with the feeling that is was, indeed, a mental defect and that did no good for her until she discovered her talent and the joy she got singing. The singer, who gained immense popularity through the show "Britain's Got Talent" realized that she had to persevere with her passions and that drove her to succeed. If a regular job is difficult to handle, then find a suitable alternative; what is important is that you persevere with what interests you and stay as independent as possible. The independence is not to achieve stardom but to lead to a happier and more contented life without feeling unnecessarily obliged to anyone.

For someone with severe seizures a home based business is ideal. Being able to work from home eliminates the stress that comes from getting to and from work when you have lost your license due to that "break through" seizure, or if you have chosen not to drive for safety reasons. It allows for flexibility when an unexpected seizure does occur and you are able to recover in a few minutes or an hour. For someone working at a "real" job, a seizure may last a minute, but well-meaning co-workers call 911, you are hauled off by ambulance to the emergency room, and you spend the rest of the afternoon getting cleared to leave. You have lost half a day of productivity that should have totaled less than two hours from start to finish. Working from home on your own terms can eliminate a lot of that. Simply put, a home-based income is a stream of income that centers the business and office in the home and does not require a 9 to 5 schedule.

The critical ingredient is getting off your butt and doing something. It's as simple as that. A lot of people have ideas, but there are few who decide to do something about them now. Not tomorrow. Not next week. But today. The true entrepreneur is a doer, not a dreamer.
–Nolan Bushnell, Entrepreneur

There are many different ways of earning an income from home. These range from having a true home based business in the spirit of the creation and shipping of a physical product (art, writing, a website) or one of the many multi-level marketing companies (I have listed them later in the book) to providing a service such as medical billing, music lessons, or tutoring in your home. There are as many different avenues for creating income from home or online as you dream or create. If you can think it, chances are, you can monetize it.

My sister is a stay at home mother who teaches piano. She has learned to tap into one of her own strengths which is playing the piano and the clarinet and teaches it from her house. She has the ability to write off a portion of her mortgage as a business expense because she has a dedicated area where she teaches. Someone who has epilepsy and musical talent such as teaching an instrument or a topic can do this from their own home. Taking this to a bigger stage, that business could be grown to offer other musicians and instruments that could be taught by employing others and managing the schedule of this tutoring and teaching at a different facility. Obviously, this requires skills in setting up a business, networking to get clients, and scheduling those clients and teaching them, but it is an example of something that can be easily grown.

For someone who does not have that much business savvy, they can go online to find companies that are looking for employees to work from home. There are call centers that employ people from their homes to answer questions about products and services. Many companies hire appointment setters in this way. Telecommuting has enabled a lot of at-home opportunities. This is a great avenue for those with epilepsy since it only requires the ability to focus on a conversation and follow through with the actual setting of appointments. These may pay as an hourly position or they may pay for each appointment that is set and confirmed.

Online sales are an income generator for many people. Someone with epilepsy can learn affiliate marketing and make sales from their computer at home. There are a variety of courses available to teach you these marketing techniques. In affiliate marketing, the salesperson receives a commission for communicating about a product or service. There is a wealth of online services that give you the chance to earn a commission for promoting these products and services. Of course, marketing online does require you to have or learn some areas of the online marketing area, social media, electronic marketing, and some website knowledge. I personally know many people who have done very well with online sales and affiliate marketing. There are online courses included in the resource section that will teach you how you can be successful in this field of endeavor. It will require an investment of time and effort to learn, but the payoff can be substantial if that is what you are interested in learning and are willing to spend the time to learn.

Contracting is generally thought of in the context of building, but a very successful home business can be constructed, pardon the pun, by doing it. You need to have a skill that you can offer someone in exchange for payment. In this respect, it could be writing, web design, or database management, all done from the comfort of your home computer. When I wrote my first book, I used Fiverr.com and Elance.com to hire contractors to do the job of creating a cover and editing for me. They did this quickly and skillfully, and I have recommended them for other jobs. If you think that you have the skills in fields such as writing, creating graphic artwork, editing, and other areas of print media, head over to Elance.com and create a profile. You can also bid on other people's projects and posted jobs, and people can see your strengths and capabilities as well as examples of your work and your hourly and project rates.

Coaching and mentoring is another great way to write your own schedule. There are many online coaches and mentors that are available that work entirely from a home environment. Some things that are very profitable as a coach would be dating and relationships, business development, network marketing, sales, wealth building, and health coaching. You can become an expert in one of these areas and share your knowledge with others. There are plenty of people who can teach you about developing an online business coaching and mentoring others. Make sure you choose someone who has experience in your field and can give you great advice and guidance.

A relative newcomer to this electronic area is blogging. One business model of it begins as you build readers to your blog and, in doing so, build areas that are not free for all members. A great example is a lady I know who blogs about, of all things nutrition. She does not charge for that blog, but does charge a membership fee for a "recipe of the week". She has several hundred followers that pay a small fee each month for four recipes a month. As you build more followers to a blog, you can also get paid by advertisers that are looking for the sort of people that you are writing for. You can also begin building an email list and sending out affiliate offers to your list that are related to your blogging topic.

Another model of this is blogging for another site. You are essentially ghostwriting based on the subject of the website. This can be quite lucrative if you can get 5 or 10 writing deals going each month, but you have to network to get those opportunities. A writer I know does quite well ghostwriting blogs in his spare time and the people that contract him to write for them send him the rough idea of the blog posts they want, he researches the content, writes the posts, then emails each post back to the company to for them to load onto their webpage. His "expertise" is largely in the fact that he can take complex technical jargon and put it into a more common language that anyone can understand. In this model, you can also build up a group of contractors that work for you, so you can handle a higher volume of writing. You have created an entire business from home, all the way down to a management structure.

In keeping with the process of writing, and creating a writing income, write a book! Becoming an author has been a passive income stream for me. I learned to do it through Alicia Dunam's course "Bestseller in a Weekend". The way that I learned to write my book and utilize keywords in the title, I am still making sales each month whether I promote my book or not. Amazon's Create Space is a great place for someone who is creative to start producing books and audio and sell them online. This is nowhere near as difficult as it seems and with online publishing, you can get your message out there very quickly.

Have you ever thought about creating your own Youtube channel? You can and there are ways to monetize and to profit from this. In a nutshell, it is a little bit like the blogging; get enough followers and then generate sales from them following you. If you have a lot to say, and don't mind telling people in front of the camera, there will plenty of people who would be interested in following your channel. Sticking a lot of people on a Youtube channel will require you to learn the ins and outs of it, but there are courses available for this type of marketing. There are plenty of online courses for Youtube marketing. I've included a couple in the resource section. You can get plenty of free tips on marketing through Youtube itself.

> *The way to get started is to quit talking and start doing.*
> –Walt Disney

The benefits to home employment are many. There is no transportation issue to be concerned with (and besides, we are not having to smell exhaust fumes which may help us out, too!). A seizure need not jeopardize your ability to get to and from work. Having a seizure at home also means you may be able to get back to work quickly, as you have plenty of flexibility in your hours. Since your office is right there in the home, you are eligible to write off some of the expense of that home if you have dedicated space to your office. Other tax advantages are also there for owning your own business, as we have covered earlier. As always, talk with your Offensive Line to help you in this. A great advantage that is there with the home based business is that you are there, not stuck on a train or commuting, with your family. The flexibility of spending time with the family when you need to cannot be stressed enough. When we feel happier, we are healthier. Our emotions are entwined with our health.

With all this upside, surely there is a downside? Of course there is. You live at work. Your office is right there, looking at you, reminding you that there are projects to be done, deadlines to meet. You have to be disciplined to stay at work and to stay off work. Family distractions may reduce your ability to be productive if you let them. Make sure you set up a way to deal with any distractions so you can remain productive.

A very real concern also has to be that you are limited in your interactions with people on a daily basis. There are some huge benefits to being "out" in the workplace, helping to dispel myths about epilepsy by being a great employee. Interacting with other people is an essential part of keeping yourself motivated and happy. It can be difficult to interact with others if you are working from home and may not have access to social activities outside your immediate neighborhood due to transportation issues. Social media and phone conversations are great, but they are no replacement for person to person interaction. This lack of social interaction can lead to loneliness and depression if the network of friends and supporters is weak or lacking. Of course, as we have seen, that strong network is also necessary to gain more opportunities for business, too. So, if you are entertaining the idea of working from home, make sure you have embraced the network and teambuilding ideas I laid out earlier in this book so you are actively getting out, networking and socializing.

The main reason people fail at home employment is because they are inconsistent and not persistent in their actions. You need to start and end each day on schedule. Draw it out and plan it the day before; calls, emails, production, sales, training, whatever it is. Schedule it! Schedule lunch, breaks, snacks, everything. This consistency will help immeasurably when you do have a seizure, because you know right where you are and right where you need to be. We all know that consistency for a person with seizure disorders can be a problem, so that schedule can help you stay on track. I know every time I have had a seizure, it feels like my brain needs to rewire itself. I feel like I have taken a step backwards. It can be very difficult to get back on track, but I can look at my gameplan for the day and know right where to be. With a little effort, my daily plan is right back in reach.

Not every home business is going to be interesting or exciting or initially, maybe even profitable. There is always a learning curve, and it can take a while for you to master the concepts needed to make money in that field. If you are working online, you may not have spent or invested the time to get a clear picture of how to be successful online. Getting found when you are online can be a tricky business as well. Get a mentor and invest some time and money into your education.

> *Any time is a good time start a company.*
> –S. V. Angel

Speaking of investments, if it is your business and you haven't done it in the past, there are investments you should make in terms of starting, learning, and running the business. These are simply the costs of being in business. Think of it as an investment in yourself. You did not have them when you worked for someone else. They handled those costs. As you build your business plan, you will incur these costs. Look for opportunities on Craigslist, Elance.com, or anywhere else we have discussed to learn more about the "how" and "how much". No matter what you think it will cost, you will need to plan on more, so make sure you are set up for startup. Spending time marketing yourself and connecting with clients before the "big jump" will help you in the startup phase.

That's right. This business investment might take money. How much? That's hard to say. Grant Cardone, sales coach and all around sharp business man, tells us in his book, "The 10X Rule" that we should plan to work ten times harder, spend ten times more money, and take ten times longer to get a new business venture started. He also points out that we will have ten times more success because we worked so hard to get it. While we are creating this business that will eventually help the economy in general and ours specifically, where can we get that money? There are some great places, but the best ones are at home, with family and friends. Speak with them about your goals for the business. They will certainly give you feedback about your plan, good or bad. This can help you refine your plan and they may donate to the cause; they may know and recommend others who will as well. You can then use this refined plan to go online to do some crowdfunding in order to help fund your project. This is essentially a venture capital idea on a small scale. People loan you money to build a business in exchange for a small percentage of ownership or the repayment of the loan. Crowdsourcing can also be useful, as you can locate people with the skills you may need for a business venture that otherwise you would have trouble locating or otherwise procuring. Sites such as Kickstarter.com and Gofundme.com can help you raise the money that you need to fund your business. Launching a crowdfunding campaign is also a great way to get the word out about your business and build excitement. Not only will you be able to gauge other's interest in the business, you will be able to connect with future clients and target markets as people share the links with their friends.

Traditional startup methods still work. Approach family and friends as investors in the company you are building. Visit the bank and apply for a small business loan. Credit cards can provide you with access to cash you may need right then, but you need to watch balances carefully and make sure you pay balances down as soon as possible so as not to incur extra expenses. As always, network! Find other business owners and learn how they funded their startup. Spend the time to learn from their mistakes and bring them into your network.

Once you have crafted your plan of action, stick with it! Make sure that every day you are taking a step towards that goal. When you start procrastinating and skipping days when working towards the goal, forgive yourself and get back on track. A great idea is to have an accountability partner to help you continually progress towards your goal – whether that is creating a business, finding the right job, or simply getting an extra part time job to meets your basic needs. With more support you will have more success.

Passive Income Creation

My rich Dad taught me to focus on passive income creation and spend my time acquiring the assets that provide passive or long term residual income... passive income from capital gains, dividends, residual income from business, rental income from real estate, and royalties.
–Robert Kiyosaki

So if I told you that there were ways to create income with no extra long term effort, would you be will to listen? Of course you would. That is passive income. A great example is my book Seizure Free, which was my first source of passive income. Even if I don't promote it, people are still purchasing it each month, since it solves a problem for them. So every month, I get a check on the royalties from the book sales. In the book I speak plainly about natural health remedies and health promoting activities that I feel contribute to me being ... Seizure Free. People buy the book and I get credit for it financially.

Other sources of passive income would include the creation of other types of products such as a CD or DVD that someone would buy, stock dividends, real estate rental income, etc... There are many ways to create a passive or residual income stream, and they all do it with little active management.

We can group these into two very broad categories, "built" or "bought". With the residual income of a "built" product, you created that product. I have already given the example of my book, but it could be a musical recording, a piece of software, anything that can be done once and then resold. It will require the effort of learning something about how to do it, then how to publicize it, but the fact is that it can continue to sell online for, literally, years, and you do not have to manage the actual product anymore. In the area of books, I must give a lot of credit to Alicia Dunam's course Bestseller in a Weekend if you have been toying with the idea of writing a book and getting it marketed. By creating things that do not need to be done again, you have created that passive income stream. Authors and musicians are great examples and if you can take the time (and have the talent) to learn how that industry works, you can stream your income, or at least a portion of it, passively.

The other main passive income stream is "bought", and by this, I mean stocks, real estate, and other physical things which pay out a residual/passive income as a result of ownership. We have all heard of "playing" the stock market. For someone who has the knowledge to be able to create an income selling and trading ownership and options, it can be a tremendous financial advantage. Buying, holding, then potentially trading stocks while earning dividends off of that companies' earnings can be a wonderful income strategy. Of course, to utilize this strategy, you need a brokerage account, the knowledge about how to buy and sell stocks and the more common mutual funds, and the money to get started. Obviously, I cannot help but recommend that you spend time with a professional financial planner to understand the nuances of the game, because you are playing with real money. Once again, members of your networking groups may be able to offer advice and a direction to base your start.

Ownership of income producing properties is another passive income stream. We have a tendency to think only in terms of rental homes or apartments, but very solid (and usually less risky) income can be produced in office and commercial spaces. Your tenants will be paying the mortgage on the property while paying rent. Of course, purchasing the property below market value is smartest, and by factoring in what the market will charge for the rental of that unit, you calculate how to keep reserves of cash for repairs, the cash needed to pay the debt servicing, and another portion that will provide you with income. There are a variety of ways to use other people's properties to pay for the initial cost of the property, and of course, once again, you start this process in your network. Learn about the local market from real estate professionals, talk to property managers (both residential and commercial) about the business and how their company works, and start looking for opportunities. Also consider using a property management company to handle the real estate in question. They will take a fee for it, but they already have their own tern network of contractors to handle work and emergencies when they arise.

Finding real estate properties, whether residential or commercial, purchasing them with someone else's money, and then renting them out to create cash flow can take a considerable amount of time. A property may be found in a month, purchased in two to three months, and may not rent for a year. You may have substantial and costly modifications to make to the structure to bring it up to the current building code. It is a slower process, but the long term asset creation is substantial.

Another often forgotten way to create passive income is Multi-Level-Marketing (MLM). Without a doubt, we see these most

Epilepsy Empowerment • 103

commonly in such common businesses as Mary Kay, Amway, and Avon, but there are literally hundreds of these companies out there, all offering a lively passive income stream. They are of derided by those who don't take the time to learn them as "pyramid schemes", but those are illegal and MLM is most certainly not!

Essentially, MLM companies work like this. You sign up as a customer, find that the products are useful to you, then become a salesperson for the company. As you build your customer base, you then sign them up as distributors under you, and you push yourself up the, for want of a better word, pyramid. The higher you go, the higher your compensation. We are all familiar with the pink Cadillacs of Mary Kay, but Arbonne (a distributor of health and wellness items) will put you in a white Mercedes if you work up their system.

Exploring this system, you need to find out how long the steps usually take. There are a lot of people that are only one or two steps up in the pyramid who may not be making money at the "job", merely getting discounts on the products that they were going to using anyway. People new to this business have a tendency to start very strong, then fade quickly when they are not rich or in a new car in six months. You need to talk to the person that is driving the car, so to speak. They will want you to be motivated and will also be invested in the business, so their advice is usually excellent.

Along the lines of the MLM idea is that of selling services that will pay you a residual each month. In this category may be included certain insurances, credit card processing sales, and monthly magazine or online subscriptions. We already touched on blog writing earlier, and this is the logical extension of that, but in the others, you may be considered a contractor for the company and paid strictly on production. You then are able to set your schedule as your health allows. The premise is very simple, you sell an individual or a merchant the service in question for an upfront fee and a set time. You will receive a commission on that sale, and then a small amount each month while the customer uses that service. If they cancel before a certain time, you will be charged some amount due to the cancellation (called a charge-back). If you can build rapport with customers and make sure that they are satisfied, then you can create a very steady income stream from these types of sales.

Now, in all of these scenarios, you can just go out there and do it with no help. And fail. I am a huge fan of coaching and mentoring. You will learn the mistakes made by others, you can understand what the issues are in the business at that time and historically, and you can do it much faster than by learning it by the seat of your pants. Most of us do not have a big bucket of money to lose on the learning curve. I have repeated in each case where these mentors can be found, and you need to find that coach to help guide you.

MLM actually comes with a coach. As a home based strategy, the person "up the line" is your coach, and you have resources directly above you at every step. The catch is simply to shop around before you sign up because you want to know that the person above you has "bought in" to the business and is as interested in success as you are. Don't just grab on to the first amazing product that you find. You want the people above you be able to guide you through the steps of acquiring clients, recruiting team members, and running your aspect of the business. You may need some additional coaching in online marketing to be able to grow your business to the next level. MyLeadSystemPro.com is an excellent resource for network marketers who want to learn how to recruit online and it is relatively inexpensive with plenty of positive support.

Finding a great coach will help you to gain focus, direction, and they will be someone who not only believes in you and your business ideas, they will be someone to hold you accountable. Oftentimes we are our own worst enemies and we begin to worry about the wrong thing. These apprehensions keep us from forging ahead and building what we know how to do. A coach and mentor can help you overcome some of these obstacles that you see and put others into perspective.

Sometimes you just can't get one out of your network, so there are actually online mentors that can teach you how to quickly sell products through webinars and also ways to create your own business online. This model is a great one to use for someone creating a business at home, but what about being the person doing the teaching? To use this to create a passive income, you need to find a product that has a monthly charge, such as a subscription service that will pay an affiliate commission. You will then need to find a reputable service that will allow you to become an affiliate of theirs. A great many products and services are out there, look for the phrase "become an affiliate" at the top or the bottom of the webpage. Amazon has even begun to allow the promotion of products and the use of an affiliate based commission. For an online passive income though, you should stick with an online subscription type of service that you can promote. This is something that can be created quickly, but the skills necessary are still going to have to be learned. You will set the pace on how much time you take to learn and implement these strategies. Remember that Youtube idea a few chapters ago? You can be a star by tying some of these differing ideas together. Become an expert and become an affiliate, and then monetize all aspects of the message!

Creating this income stream is going to be anything but passive. It will require massive action and you will need to invest tremendous amounts of time and energy in the beginning. There are many advantages to having this passive income, though, and without a doubt, one of the most important is for when you are incapacitated. When seizures are overwhelming you due to changes in your medicines, having that passive stream is a Godsend. You don't worry about driving to work. You have a way to pay for medical expenses. You have folding money in hand! Passive income will help you stay afloat when you are not feeling your best and give you something to help you build real wealth.

Heroes

I have researched and studied the effects of epilepsy, the medications, and the treatments for years, trying to find ways to limit the effect the disorder had on my life. In that time, I have met many people who continue to inspire me as I move through and conquer this affliction. We have talked about big names that everyone knows, such as Julius Caesar or FloJo, but the real heroes are the men and women who overcome epilepsy and are not famous. They get up, go to work, add value to the lives of friends and family, and are inspirational to me because in many ways, their stories are about a real life. I challenge you to look for people that are doing this in your world, and I challenge you to be one of them. The first one of these heroes is Stephen Pirokowski. This is a part of his story, and I hope you can see why I find him so inspiring.

When I was two years old, the German measles were brought to my house. After a short time, I got encephalitis and an incredibly high fever, the end result of which was scarring on my brain. It was this scarring that caused me to have seizures. Until the fourth grade, I suffered from petit mal seizures, which also caused me to be held back in the third grade. I spent a great deal of time in the principal's office because my teachers all thought I was a daydreamer. That year there was a teacher at the school who was a little more learned about things, and she encouraged my parents to take me to a neurologist.

I still remember that first trip to see the neurologist; a man came into the waiting area in a wheelchair, and in the course of the conversation, he volunteered to me and my parents that he was in a wheelchair because of encephalitis, the same thing that I had suffered from. I was terrified.

The doctor, as always, prescribed a medication to help with the seizures, and I HATED taking it. I mean, me and this anticonvulsant? Hate at first sight. I would try to spit it out, and you know how that went down with my family. I guess you could say that I took enough of it through my teenage years, but I couldn't stand it. As a teenager, of course, there were always those kids in the school who stayed up all night, took drugs, partied a lot. I would look at them the next day, hungover, coming down from the high, and I began to wonder if they felt the way I did after I would have a seizure. Some of them described it in some of the same language that I would have used, so I began to go a read up and try to figure out what caused my seizures. I found that regular exercise had been linked to the release of endorphins in the brain, and that those endorphins often made you feel better. I began to jog regularly, and I found that running not only made me stronger, it actually helped to control my seizures.

So, flash forward to age thirty, the rebellious little kid spitting out his medicine is running all the time and he is running marathons. I ran the New York marathon first, then I ran all the big ones in the United States. New York, Boston, Chicago, you name it. If it was 26.2 miles, I tried to get there to run it.

Then something else happened. Life. I became a father, adopting twins from Hungary. I took off my running shoes and put on my Daddy Hat. My doctor had seen that my seizures were under control, so my medication was long gone, and that was when I began to have seizures again. I was staying at home with the lads, not getting the exercise that I had become used to, and I started right back with the seizures. What could I do? I had a full time job taking care of them, so I was back to living with it. Being a dad is great, be an epileptic again wasn't. Finally when my boys were about eight, I began to run again, and I saw the seizures lessen, then disappear.

Never forget that life does not stop because you are having a bad day. I divorced, I moved back to New York State. I had grown up in New Jersey, and like so many people living in the shadow of New York City, I had worked all around that area. When I was going to Brookdale College, I had worked in a print shop. The owners were good people, I had told them I had seizures occasionally, and they could not have been nicer about it. One day, I had a real doozie, hit my head and burned the side of my face badly when I hit a radiator. They gave me the week off, even when I told them I didn't need it, I wanted to work. Later on in school, I helped to set up self-help groups on campus, for epilepsy and other organizations, but I could really get behind the epilepsy one. I felt like we had a great opportunity since so many of us that couldn't drive could get around with public transportation. The really neat part of the group was that we swapped venues. We might meet here on day, then the next meeting would be at somebody's house. By doing it that way, we could all share the burden of transportation, and no one specific person had it any better or worse than anyone else.

Anyhow, I told you that to tell you this, I have worked all sorts of jobs, but I have always loved to cook. I was very fortunate to land a job when my boys were about six months old with a wealthy family in Manhattan, down in one of the richest neighborhoods in the city. I worked for them, and they didn't mind if I moonlighted a little, so I built a small catering business. I had plenty of other jobs, with my own family to provide for, my seizures to deal with, we have heard all the excuses. In the end, though, I really wanted to cook. I just loved it.

While my wife and I were on our honeymoon out of the country, I had had a couple of seizures, then I was fortunate to get the treatment I needed. When I got back to the United States, I had two more seizures, and I began to look around for what kind of help might be out there for me. I was a long way past school age, and I found a program in New York called Adult Career and Continuing Education Services – Vocational Rehabilitation, or, as everyone calls it, ACCES/VR. They actually helped to fund me going to school at the French Culinary Institute. It is a great program for the person that is not afraid to work hard at their personal growth and education and keep at it. They expect you to be successful.

I'm in the second year of school there, and it has been amazing. For the first year, I made the President's list two consecutive semesters. I was appointed to be a mentor to other students who are having problems. I am trying to show them that there is always a way to be a better student and to gain the skills you need for the course and use the knowledge from the course in the real world. I have also gotten a part-time job on campus working for and with students that have disabilities in the college. Ten hours each week, I help to arrange accommodations for them in and outside the campus. The amount of confidence that all this has given me, plus being in the second year program, I feel that I can be placed into any kitchen and produce top results for an employer or a professor. As an example, one of the classes I'm taking is American Baking. I won't go into why that is so different from Greek Baking, but you get my drift. This course also supplies the dining room with all the desserts for lunch and dinner. I have taken courses on menu planning, nutrition, really all aspects of cooking.

I have always had to work harder than other students because of my memory problems, and it has changed the way that I study. I found an App for my phone called Quizlet, so I study while I travel. I am on the bus for about two hours, since I don't drive (and who wants to in the Big Apple?) so I study chapters in the program anywhere I travel. I have actually written the last few courses I have had and I share that with other students as a sort of "real world" version that they can see not only the "how" but also the "why". I know I learn by repetition, and a lot of others do, r even got outside for a five minute break. This year, I am still studying like crazy, but I've learned how to study better for me.

Oh, yeah, I have started back running. I have made well over four thousand miles this year, and worn out a pair or two of Nikes. My message is not about me, it is so much more than that. For whatever reason, these things in my life are all mine. My success is, in the end, going to be judged on how well I aligned them to make the most out of everything given to me, whether I see those things as good or bad. I have chosen to see them as all good.

～

Alexander Lodi is a blogger who has suffered from epilepsy since the first year of his life. He currently blogs and is a member of the Epilepsy Foundation. Alexander's blog is epilepsymentor.com. He is helping people to create a positive life despite having a chronic condition and providing resources for others with epilepsy. He has links on his blog for people to help them to work from home with epilepsy and build a career of value.

I had acquired epilepsy at the age of one. It was an allergic reaction to pertussis vaccine. I ran a very high fever of 106 degrees. They actually quit taking my temperature, it was so high. I was burning up. From that point on, I started getting seizures like an epileptic. I've had it for 46 years now. It has certainly created a lot of auras but I rarely get anything like a big, drop down, Grand Mal seizure. My type of epilepsy is known as Temporal Lobe Epilepsy, which, I'm sure you know, is the most common form. I have had it for 46 years and have really been able to get along well and even drove up until December of 2007. Getting along with people in school was tough because I stereotyped myself as someone that was not going to be accepted. So, of course, I kept to myself. In the process of keeping to myself, I came across as being better than other people. You tend to be disliked in school, then you keep your guard up the rest of your life. Dating was a challenge because I feared rejection.

I came out of my shell about epilepsy back in 2007. I had moved back home after having a Grand Mal seizure while driving. I didn't know what had happened. I was driving, then I was parked, then I came to and my partner was driving. Going to work the next morning, I had another one and crashed into a tree. So from that point on, I said, "no more driving." I did not want to put anyone's life on the line because of my vanity. That's where I actually started talking about it. I started online with Facebook and then I got my blog out there. I started supporting people and the Epilepsy Foundation. As you talk about it, it becomes easier to talk about. You can see that you are making a difference in other people's lives.

Sharing with others made me realize that the acceptance from them was always there. Nobody had ever rejected me because I had seizures. I just wasn't willing to put myself out there. Since I put it out there, nobody has rejected me.

I made a very good friend from the Epilepsy Foundation and she had a really bad time around Christmas a few years ago. She came up and spent the week with us and we talked a lot. We talked about epilepsy, about the medication, about feeling like a zombie because of the medicines, and about just feeling lost and disconnected. All I could do is just support her. I didn't feel like I did anything special, but I was speechless when later, on the telephone, she told me how much I had helped her. I felt verbally validated that I, or could, help just by being a good listener.

For the person who has just started to have seizures, I would say this: Write down a list of your dreams and never give up on them no matter what anyone says. Epilepsy is not a roadblock at all. If anything, it is a way to reach out and help others with that type of a condition. It does not define you, nor does it make you somehow less of a person. Too many epileptics try to keep it to themselves, bury it down deep, and pretend that it somehow isn't there. It is, but it is not the defining characteristic of an individual.

Live your life to the fullest! I'm a goal setter, which is very important. You can never give up. Don't listen to the naysayers, keep moving forward and find like-minded people. Having a goal and working towards it can really help to keep you focused and driven.

I can't help but talk about how my outlook has improved as a result of finding God and growing in my Faith. We all have bad days; when I have a bad day, I go inside myself and I pray. I open up my Bible. I even have an app on my iPod and I'll read a little bit of the Bible on it each day. If you read and follow my blog, you'll see that I've had four angelic experiences, the first of which included my mother coming back to see me. I even have one about being carried by God. I have learned the power of being positive and coupling that with Faith. It is so very powerful.

∽

What follows is the very interesting story of Guy W. Stoker, who was driven to research epilepsy and some of its rarer forms. His has had it his whole life, but it has also helped to provide purpose in his whole life. He was kind enough to lend a few pages to my book to show that epilepsy need not control you, you can derive direction and assist the study and still do something that you love...

My name is Guy R. Stoker. I have had Right Frontal-Temporal Lobe Epilepsy since birth, which was exacerbated from the age of 11 following head injuries and other issues, though my epilepsy was not diagnosed until the age of 27.

Throughout the years my seizures manifested themselves in a variety of ways from Absence Seizures through Tonic-Clonic Seizures with Complex Partial and TEA Seizures in the mix. The big issues in my case were that for many years most of my seizures would manifest at night, and also in cases where I was taken to the hospital, none of the tests showed anything at all, including EEG, Sleep Deprived EEG, MRI. fMRI, and CAT scans. This was a very difficult period as I was living with a condition that I had no name for. My family and I were sure it was epilepsy, but there was no hard clinical evidence to back it up, and therefore I wasn't being offered any treatment. It was only in early 2003 when I was in the hospital for a completely unrelated issue and had a seizure witnessed by a senior consultant neurologist that I finally had a name for what I had lived with for the past 27 years, Epilepsy.

This diagnosis was a double edged sword as it meant I finally knew what it was and they could finally start trying to find the right treatment, but during this period, I had to surrender my driving license which I felt as a major blow to my independence and to my work prospects as a professional musician. I became dependent on family, friends, and other musicians to be able to work as a musician, which significantly reduced the level of work I could do outside of my main job which was teaching music and performing arts in secondary school. At that time I had not been made aware of the free bus travel or disabled persons rail pass which were available to me, though as a pianist/keyboard player would have made no difference, as they are very un-portable instruments in comparison to others such as guitar or similar wind instruments. The loss of my driving license obviously had a big impact on my personal and social life, too.

After much consideration, of various issues, such as the local job market, my ambitions, my health, and opportunities, I decided to return to studies, and to pursue a Masters degree in Contemporary

Composition at Dartington College of Arts (UCF) UK, starting in September of 2008. As part of my study in 2009 I attended the first International Conference on Music and Emotion at Durham University. Following this line of study on my return to Dartington, in McDonald Critchley's book Music & the Brain (1977) I came across a rare form of Temporal Lobe Epilepsy called Musicogenic Seizures which are cases of the patients' emotional response to a particular sound, song, or a piece of music manifesting as a seizure. Dr. Peter W. Kaplan (JHU) wrote a paper on this condition in 2003. In his paper he refers to the case of a young Japanese girl in 2001, whose only seizure trigger was the song "Happy Birthday."

Following further research including a visit in October 2009 to Johns Hopkins University Hospital (JHU) in Baltimore, MD, I was invited to co-write a paper on this form of seizure with Dr. Peter W. Kaplan for a conference on Epilepsy, Brain, & Mind, in Prague 2010. At the conference session on Epilepsy in the Arts, the session was led by the world leading expert in this field Dr. Steven C. Schachter (Harvard) who invited me to explore the use of music as a means of nonverbal expression of the experience of living with epilepsy, and present my findings in Rome, 2011. This was an enormous and unique invitation and opportunity as it allowed me to bring together the two biggest parts of my life, music and epilepsy. This exploration resulted in my successful completion of my MA, including the composition of the album Ictal Variations (A Musical Exploration of Epilepsy) which has since gone on to feature in conference speeches, international epilepsy arts exhibitions including Hidden Truths Project (CA) in 2013 and 2014, and my dissertation, An Investigation in to the place of Music in the field of Epilepsy Arts (Stoker, 2010) extracts of which have been published in medical journals. The album has helped me and many other people with and without epilepsy to gain a better understanding of the diversity of the condition, and those who live with it. The interrelationship between music and epilepsy in various contexts continues to be the basis of my work today, and through this opportunity I have learnt a huge amount about the condition I'm living with, come across some amazing works, and met some truly remarkable people. So for this I say thank you to Dr. Kaplan, Dr. Schachter, my family and friends for their continuous love and support, and, in a strange sort of way, thank you epilepsy.

∽

Some people are remarkable and uplifting just through their comments on epilepsy and the actions they take to show it is not a hurdle to success. I first learned about Jamie Simon in one of the many Facebook groups I frequent. I have encouraged her to share some of her story with us because of the uplifting advice she was showing by example and giving others. I was surprised to learn that she had gone to the Special Olympics and medaled four times!

My name is Jamie Simon and I live in Cache Bay, Ontario, Canada. I have had epilepsy for three years, but I have never let it stop me. I decided I have no choice but to be positive so it will not slow me down one bit. I went to the Special Olympics and have won 4 gold medals, 3 at the Provincials in Vaughn, Ontario and 1 at the Nationals in Vancouver, British Columbia. I do not let this control my life, because if I do, I will lose out on living my life. I have learned the hard way, but in life, you can and must do the things you want.

Look at me, I am a success story. You can do the same thing with your own "can-do" attitude and positive thinking; just say to yourself that you can do it. We all have to choose a way, my way is with a positive attitude.

For any questions and answers and to connect with Jamie Simon go to simonjamie76@yahoo.com. She is an awesome person.

My Story

Long ago I learned that living with the diagnosis of a long term chronic disease is an extremely daunting task. Being forced to accept a host of side effects and huge medication costs can be a gateway to depression and a rash of alternate health problems that can swing the sufferer into the downward spiral of mental trauma as well as physical. As I got older, I began to look for other ways to find healing from epilepsy, but it took many years to get there. I have learned that alternative medicines can be amazingly empowering and healing.

Now, this is not to say that my family shunned modern Western medicine. At the ripe old age of seven, I noticed that I wheezed a lot during physical activity. I was taken to the doctor and they determined that I had asthma when the wheezing did not stop. The doctor we went to see gave me an inhaler, taught me and my mother how I was to use it, and I was back to running around like every other seven year old in the world. I actually felt validated and quite grown up for understanding why I had been so slow running around the track during PE and I honestly felt pretty special because I had my trusty inhaler to help me breath, just in case.

The down side of the inhaler was that it never really seemed to be all that effective in clearing my airways. There were many times when I felt that just the act of slowing down my breathing to use the inhaler was more useful than the paltry atomized mix of medicine and air that it shot into my lungs. Seasonal allergies began to trigger my asthma and before long, I was seeing an allergist for shots on a regular basis. Despite the shots, I always liked my allergist; he had a great sense of humor, and despite some seasonal sneezing, my parents and I figured that as long as I wasn't going to the hospital because I couldn't breathe, we were doing better than before.

Flash forward to the age of thirteen. I had started having seizures "out of the blue" and after a barrage of tests, they determined it was epilepsy. I remember asking the doctor why I suddenly had this disorder, and his answer was pretty telling. "It is idiopathic. That means we're idiots and we really don't know how or why you have it." I loved his quick wit, and I looked up to him for that sort of honesty. He seemed to care about me as a person, and my parents and I just accepted that the anticonvulsants that he had to prescribe were going to damage my liver. This neurologist just felt that this was a fact of life with epilepsy and it was something that we could monitor. Hindsight being what it is, there really was never a point when we discussed what we would do when a liver function test came back to show that I could no longer stay on that medication. Truth be told, my neurologist never really went over liver function tests with us or dwelled on the idea very much at all.

So I went off into anticonvulsant land and they really didn't work very well at first. I had to up my dosage every few weeks. It felt like we were guessing and checking with each dose and added medication. Finally, my doctor recommended that I see an endocrinologist. I got poked and prodded, and finally, diagnosed at the age of 14 with Hashimoto's Thyroiditis. This is an autoimmune disease where the thyroid gland is actually attacked by the antibodies in the body and leads to a whole host of potential issues. The irony was that I had none of the symptoms other than testing low on the series of tests they had given me. The endocrinologist prescribed Synthroid (a synthetic version of the hormones that I was low on) and I had to take it once a day. I remember how sweet it tasted on my tongue before I swallowed it, and, years later, I wonder if it was really just a sugar pill. My parents were convinced, though, that this was another part of the key to my seizure control as the seizure control stabilized after adding Synthroid. To the credit of the doctors, I did not have seizures for several years after this treatment regimen began.

I got along to get along through high school, but the costs of the medicines were outrageous. When I graduated high school, I inherited about a thousand dollar a month set of medical costs due to the prescriptions and hefty insurance bills, and of course, I was told that generics could not be substituted, since some random ingredient in the generic might trigger a seizure. At this point, I guess I still believed in what the doctors told me, so I kept on. Of course, I also learned that for someone with a preexisting condition, health insurance was prohibitively high.

I went through that silliness for well over a decade. During that time, I had become increasingly interested in fitness, and I had learned many different things about physical health and wellness. I had also learned a lot about medicine as it is practiced in the Far East and in the Western world. The truth of the matter is that in the so-called "developed" world, you can get tossed from specialist to specialist and very few of them actually talk to each other.

As an example, let's say you have congestive heart failure, you live in a major American city, and you have several other health issues. The hospital is going to keep you alive via machine, cardiologists will pump you full of medication to help solve the issues with your heart, but when your kidneys start to fail, they may not speak at all to the specialists that are brought in to solve your renal issues. This will result in another round of medications that may or may not interact properly with the ones "helping" your heart, and all the while, your liver is taking a beating. You can't die, since you're tied to a machine, but your quality of life is in the toilet.

Well-meaning family are being given "living" options that do not take into account what kind of life you may have if you make it out of the hospital at all. The medical bills pile up, and all these specialists are still not talking to one another. This lack of a simple face-to-face conversation with the patient and the team of doctors has become the standard in the West. We have forgotten to take into account the quality of life and the desire for life. Better yet, we have not taken into account how to prevent the cardiac event from occurring in the first place. A lifetime spent seeking good health practices can eliminate an issue like this at the end of it.

This lack of communication with the different doctors I personally dealt with drove me to look at ways I could actively assist MY health. I researched the nutritional deficiencies we have as sufferers of epilepsy and I started exercising regularly. Prescription drugs were wreaking havoc on my health and my body – I routinely had double vision, muscle aches, depression. The final straw was when my hair fell out.

I had gone to a dermatologist who prescribed a steroid to regrow my hair and the next month was my yearly visit to my endocrinologist. He was unable to test my blood due to the steroid I was taking, so I had to come off the steroids for the blood test to be valid. So I went off the steroid, the hair that grew back fell out, and I was right back where I had started. The steroids had regrown my hair, but I was fat and the smooth, beautiful skin I had had my whole life was breaking out with acne. I finally decided that it wasn't worth it, and I would solve this issue on my own; I had found the courage to start taking action. The words of that neurologist long ago came back to me … "we're idiots and we really don't know…"

I started off with some very basic diet ideas. In the previous years, I had read many books on diet, from the blood type diet, the Paleo, Adkins, low-carb, even the Gut and Psychology Syndrome

Diet. I was fascinated with the idea that I could control my health with simple food and exercise. After trying a few different diets, I settled on the basic idea of eliminating processed foods and increasing my vegetable intake.

As for the exercise, I have already discussed my love of swimming, and at that time, I was a swim instructor. As I explored my health options and opportunities, I learned other exercise disciplines, such as Pilates, and different ways to stretch to improve your posture. I learned that good posture was a key ingredient in good breathing, and as my body became healthier and my posture improved, my asthma was eliminated. I began to realize that I could recognize symptoms early and correct any breathing issue I created.

I had done things to improve my posture, but I had several breakthroughs in that area by visiting a chiropractor. My mother had taken me from time to time when I was a teenager for my spine (there was that posture thing again) and once, the chiropractor had given me an adjustment that cleared up the congestion in my head in a matter of minutes. This incident helped to inspire me to look outside of "conventional" medicine for answers to the many questions I had begun to ask.

In all this living research, I had met many new friends that opened up doors and ideas to me about supplements and vitamins that could help me in my search for better health. This in turn led me to alternate healers and practitioners who opened other doors into health for me. I did figure out that a person can spend an awful lot of money to cure themselves of a chronic illness by unconventional means, but that the journey back to "normal" was well worth it.

As I said previously, I began a routine to correct my posture, and as I did that and researched the health benefits of it, I came across the Buteyko breathing method. Buteyko felt that the root cause of many diseases and ailments was improper breathing and thus, a lack of oxygen. As the research has come along, his theories have been validated, and his belief in the strength of nasal breathing and the correct volume of each breath have changed the way many people do this most common of exercises. Due to our modern lifestyle, we do not breathe with our diaphragm through our noses, and this causes our brains and bodies to function at less than a nominal rate. I started to breathe through my nose and immediately noticed some improvements in how I felt. This was such a simple thing to improve and in the end, the improvements were tremendous. As I focused more and more on proper breathing, I started to taper off my medication. I was nervous that oxygenation was not my only problem, but I was willing to try. Completely free of the anticonvulsant, I averaged a seizure once every few months. This was the same result that the medications had! I was restoring my health through proper breathing, quality foods, and exercise.

So I felt great, but my hair had still not come back, and in the course of researching ways to improve my thyroid condition, I read about the theories of Dr. Batmangheli. His idea was simple. You aren't sick, you're thirsty. The human body starts to break down when it doesn't get enough water. This water helps to cleanse the body through the more active elimination of waste and success had been reported with allergies, asthma, and even lupus. Drinking half my body weight in ounces each day with the addition of sea salt to keep minerals I needed in my body caused my skin to clear up and my hair began to come back.

The real shock was realizing that seizures can be a sign of dehydration. All this time, I could have been drinking water instead of a weird mix of pills that cost a fortune. The solution seemed almost too simple. I began to see health improvements over time. My body began to be feel even healthier. My skin improved. I never use lotion. I had fewer coughs and sneezes.

I now believe that asthma, which affects 14 million children and kills thousands each year, is really a complication caused by dehydration in the body. Asthma limits the free passage of air from the blood cells to the lungs due to this drought at the cellular level. Recognizing these issues in the asthmatic and taking the steps necessary to change them can help millions and begin to reverse the damages caused by asthma.

Improving my health has really been a lifelong journey. Hundreds of hours of research, thousands of dollars wasted on medications that did nothing to help and a lot to hurt me, and years of thinking I was somehow inferior to others due to obscure conditions led me to the conclusions in this book. As for the medications for my thyroid? I quit taking them long ago as I rebuilt my body. I have lived the life I outline in this book, and it has worked for me. My advice IS this book. Epilepsy has stopped millions over the course of human history. It very nearly stopped me. I now know that we, collectively, can stop it. Do I think that every single person suffering from epilepsy can become seizure free? I think so. There will always be exceptions, people that have egregious health conditions or other issues that may prevent them ever being totally free, but I think that by deciding to take action, refusing to accept the very arbitrary status quo of medical experts, and empowering themselves to be healthy, a huge percentage of those suffering from epilepsy can live a more productive, happier, and healthier life. I am living the proof of it today.

Resources

Resources for Conquering Your Fear
1. Neurowisdom.com – The Neurowisdom 101 course will teach you how to retrain your mind to focus more on the positive.
2. ThinkRightNow.com – Positive affirmations CDs and computer software that will help you to change your habits by changing your thought patterns.
3. The Magic of Thinking Big by David Schwartz – An excellent book that describes the power behind our thoughts.
4. Success Through a Positive Mental Attitude by Napolean Hill – Another excellent book that shows you how to shift your mind to focus on the positive in order to create your own success.
5. Energy Healing – Tara Taglienti – Find simple ways to release negative energy though energy healing. Tara also has a blog talk radio show, The Show Up Show! Find her on facebook - https://www.facebook.com/tara.taglienti
6. The Ultimate Results Coaching – Joey Martina can coach you to help you unblock some of the things that are holding you back. http://theultimateresults.com

Resources for Job Hunting
1. Craigslist.com – Online classified search engine with local job listings. Also a resource that can be used when searching for employees for a start-up company.

2. Monster.com – Online resume and job listing site that generally focuses on lower or entry level skill positions.
3. CareerBuilder.com – Online resume and job listing site that includes a wide range of positions and skill requirements.
4. LinkedIn.com – A fantastic networking site allowing you to establish yourself and connect with people in a social media setting that is driven for the building of business networking. It will also allow you to showcase the skills that you have and your business acumen.

Resources to Obtain Funding for Your Small Business
1. Kickstarter.com – Crowdfunding for your creative projects and small businesses. Personal fundraising is not allowed.
2. Gofundme.com – Crowdfunding for personal fundraising
3. Indigogo.com – Crowdfunding site for personal and creative projects. Indigogo has a mobile app for one touch funding.
4. Teespring.com- Tee shirt crowdfunding site. Here you can create and sell tee-shirts. Here is a place to sell high quality apparel with zero up-front costs and zero risks.

Resources for Financial Aid for Those With Disabilities
1. Financial Aid for Disabled Students – http://www.finaid.org/otheraid/disabled.phtml
2. Scholarships for Students with Epilepsy – http://www.college-scholarships.org/health/epileptic-students.htm

Resources to Finding Networking and Business Opportunities
1. Business Networking International (BNI) – BNI.com BNI is the largest business networking organization in the world.

Members are highly encouraged to give referral to other members. Weekly meetings encourage participation, interaction, and success.

2. Meetup.com – An Online resource that connects you with other people who have the same interests. Many networking groups post on Meetup.com, and this could be a great place to post and start your own networking group and build a client base.
3. Evenbrite.com – Allows you to search for events by location and category. It also allows you to register for the event as well as easily share events with your connections.
4. Eventful.com – Is an events website which not only lists events, it also has a social networking aspect allowing you to connect with other users.
5. Grant Cardone – Mr. Cardone is a very experienced business man with over 30 years of sales experience. His books and videos not only provide a great model and inspiration, his insights on positive thinking and its correlation to success are very beneficial. Grantcardone.com

Resources for Online Sales and Online Selling
1. Amazon.com – The world's largest online marketplace. They have an affiliate program. You can promote any of the products that they sell on your website and earn a small commission.
2. Createspace.com – Create a product or book that can be sold on Amazon. This is a great place to start if you are new to writing and want your book available quickly.
3. KDP.com – Kindle Direct Publishing – Publishing site for Kindle ebooks. This is an easy method to get published and sell your ebook quickly on Amazon.
4. Etsy.com – A creative marketplace for people who are "crafty" to sell their wares.

5. Elance.com – An online writing site where you can post jobs and apply for jobs in the field of writing. A great resource to find editors, virtual assistants, page layout artists, and graphic designers.
6. Fiverr.com – Another online writing site where you can post for smaller projects and get paid for those skills. Typically each job is worth five dollars, hence the name.
7. Melindacurle.com/freevideomarketingcourse – A course to learn how to utilize Youtube to get started making money through affiliate marketing and online sales.

Resources for Building Your Offensive Line
1. National Society of Accountants – NSACCT.org -A great site that has a list of over 700,000 accountants available to help you narrow down who to use for your tax protection.
2. For a great place to start obtaining information about attorneys, look to the American Bar Association's website –www.americanbar.org
3. A great option for the basics of legal protection is also Legal Shield. They offer affordable legal and identity theft protection in many different areas of the law. Contact Sandra Caron (754)-800-9557 or online at www.sandracaron.legalshieldassociate.com
4. Life insurance questions are all about relationships, and the best place to start is going to be at a local agent's office. Even if you do not have life or health insurance, local property and casualty firms can often direct you to a company or local agent that can serve to educate you not only on coverage and underwriting, but also what types of policies are best. In a pinch, you can contact the gentleman we interviewed, Presley Lomax at www.presleylomax.com.

Resources for a Network Marketing Home-Based Business
1. MyLeadSystemPro.com – An online educational community to teach you how to market and recruit members online.
2. MLMInsider.com – An online resource for articles, training, meetings and press releases about the MLM business scene.
3. Catalystmlm.com – Another site that is dedicated to sharing tools and ideas for the successful marketing of many different MLM concepts.

The 100 Top MLM or Direct Sales companies, how much they are worth, and the country in which they are based-

1. Alticor (Amway) $11.3B, USA
2. Avon Products, Inc. $10.7B, USA
3. Herbalife Ltd. $4.1B, USA
4. Vorwerk Co. KG $3.3B, Germany
5. Natura Cosmeticos SA $3.2B, Brazil
6. Mary Kay, Inc. $3.1B, USA
7. Tupperware Brands Corp. $2.6B, USA
8. Nu Skin Enterprises, Inc. $2.2B, USA
9. Oriflame Cosmetics SA $2B, Luxembourg
10. Belcorp Ltd $1.9B, Peru
11. Primerica Financial Services, Inc. $1.2B, USA
12. Pola $1.2B, Japan
13. Miki Corp. $1.1B, Japan
14. Ambit Energy, L.P. $930M, USA
15. Telecom Plus $892M, UK
16. Stream Energy (Ignite) $840M, USA
17. Yanbal International $815M, Peru
18. Thirty-One Gifts, LLC $718M, USA

Epilepsy Empowerment • 131

19. Shaklee Corp. $650M, USA
20. USANA Health Services Inc. $649M USA
21. ViSalus (Blyth) $624M, USA
22. ACN, Inc. $582M, USA
23. Scentsy $560M, USA
24. Hermes $550M, Brazil
25. WIV Wein International AG $539M, Germany
26. AmorePacific $520M, South Korea
27. Market America Inc. $505m, USA
28. The Pampered Chef Ltd. $500M, USA
29. For Days Co. Ltd. $445M, Japan
30. Southwestern $427M, USA
31. PartyLite (Blyth) $425M, USA
32. KK ASSURAN $378M, Japan
33. Arbonne International LLC $377M, USA
34. Nature's Sunshine Products, Inc. $368M, USA
35. LG Household and Health Care $350M, South Korea
36. Isagenix International $334M, USA
37. Faberlic $330M, Russia
38. Neways, Inc. $326M, Japan
39. Noevir Holdings Co., Ltd, $326M, Japan
40. Menard Japan Cosmetics $319M, Japan
41. Eureka Forbes Ltd. $318M, India
42. LR Health & Beauty Systems $313M, Germany
43. Team National, Inc. $301M, USA
44. Longrich (Jiangsu Longliqi) $287M, China
45. 4Life Research L.C. $268M, USA
46. Charlie Corp. Ltd. $258M, Japan
47. Advocare International L.P. $255M USA
48. PM-International $249M, Germany
49. Ann Summers $235M, UK
50. Naturally Plus $233M, Japan

51. Team Beachbody $218M, USA
52. Take Shape For Life (Medifast) $216M, USA
53. JapanLife $215M, Japan
54. K par K $214M, France
55. Family Heritage Life $202M, USA
56. CUTCO (Vector Marketing) $200M, USA
57. Huis Clos $200M, France
58. It Works! Global $200M, USA
59. BearCere'Ju Co. Ltd. $192M, Japan
60. Hillarys Blinds $189M, UK
61. LifeVantage Corp. $187M, USA
62. KOYOSHA $186M, Japan
63. Viridian Energy $182M, USA
64. Mannatech, Inc. $173M, USA
65. Elken $172M, Malaysia
66. GNLD $170M, USA
67. Organo Gold International $170M, Canada
68. Enagic USA, Inc. $165M, USA
69. North American Power $165M, USA
70. Lux International $163M, Switzerland
71. Hy Cite Enterprises, LLC. $159M, USA
72. Princess House, Inc. $148M, USA
73. Zhulian Marketing $145M, Malaysia
74. Sportron $143M, USA
75. WorldVentures Holdings, LLC. $143M, USA
76. Nikken Global Inc. $133M, USA
77. Jeunesse Global $126M, USA
78. Univera $121M, USA
79. TriVita $120M, USA
80. Vemma Nutrition Co. $117M, USA
81. Zija International $110M, USA
82. Rodan+Fields $108M, USA

83. 5Linx Enterprises, Inc. $104M, USA
84. Momentis $103M, USA
85. The Longaberger Company $100M, USA
86. Nerium International $100M, USA
87. Akasuka $98M, Japan
88. Creative Memories $97M, USA
89. Tastefully Simple Inc. $96M, USA
90. Vision International People Group $95M, Cyprus
91. Ion Cosmetics $93M, Japan
92. Chandeal Co. Ltd. $86M, Japan
93. Nefful $79M, Japan
94. Kleeneze, Ltd. $76M, UK
95. Youngevity $75M, USA
96. The Maira Co. Ltd. $72M, Japan
97. Supreme Products $72M, Japan
98. Nature Care $71M, Japan
99. Reliv International $69M, USA
100. Zurvita $63M USA

Home Based Business Ideas

- Childcare
- Medical Billing
- Beauty Makeovers
- Accountability Coach
- ADHD Coach
- Travel Advisor/Planner
- Dating and Relationship Coach
- Matchmaker
- Acupuncture
- Advertising Consultant
- Advertising Copy Writer
- Affiliate Marketer
- Affiliate Marketing Coach
- After School Art Program
- After School Music Teacher
- Alternative Healer
- Animal Care/Per Boarding
- Appointment Coordinator
- Audio Book Reading
- Manicure/Pedicure
- Voice Lessons for Singers
- Business Strategist
- Benefits Advisor for Entrepreneurs
- Bilingual Tutor
- Birthday Party Planner
- Bookkeeping Services
- Business Coach
- Tutor Training
- Business Risk Consultant
- Organizational Coach to un-clutter homes
- Car Washing/Detailing
- Computer Consulting
- Tax Consultant
- Hair Accessories
- Cooking Coach
- Meal Planner
- Fitness Trainer – Boot Camps
- Personal Trainer
- Web-based Fitness Coach
- Dance Teacher
- Interior Decorator/Coach
- Epilepsy Mentor
- Podcaster for Parenting Advice
- Network Coordinator
- Network Mentor
- Real Estate Ebook Writer
- Real Estate Investor
- Marketing Materials Advisor
- Cleaning Service Owner
- Dog Walker
- Etiquette Coach
- Ebay/Online Sales Coach
- Ebooks Distribution
- Ebook Creation
- Recipe/Cookbook Writer
- Financial Coach

- Financial Planner
- Fashion Designer
- Fashion Consultant
- Fitness Blogger
- Ghost Write
- Grant Writer
- Gourmet Food Products
- Green Cleaning Products
- Handyman Service
- Home Party Planner
- Home repair
- Image Consultant
- Identity Theft Consultant
- Home Staging for Real Estate Sales
- Lead Generation
- Sales Trainer
- Hair Dresser
- Jewelry Repair
- Jewelry Sales
- Wedding Consultant
- Make Up Lessons on DVD
- Mentor for People with Disabilities
- Marketing Consultant
- Massage Services
- Negotiation Trainer
- MLM Nutritional Products
- Motivational Speaker
- Parenting Coach
- Online Parenting Lessons
- Cake Decorator
- Specialized Photography – weddings, etc…
- Pet Accessories
- Personal Job Hunter/ Recruiter
- Personal Assistant Services
- Remote Secretarial Services
- Promotional Products
- Property Management
- Referral Partnerships
- Revenue Model Explanations
- Seminar Leader
- Non-Profit Advisor/ Advocate
- Web Designer

Some of these may look impossible to someone that is not driving, but the answer is networking. You do not have to be the person walking the dog, you can be the person scheduling the walk and running the operation. Many of these do require previous experience, but all of us have a set of skills, many that can be used to be successful from a home-based company. By refusing to be negative and simply spending the time to look at how a business can grow, you may find that a home based business is easier than the ones that you struggled with in the so-called real world.

Using our dog walking model, let's grow that from just you and a few clients. Your business is successful, and you realize that to make the amount of money you want, you need to either walk 35 dogs a day at the current rate or you need to charge $30 per dog. Since no one is going to pay $30 to have their dog walked, and you physically cannot walk 35 dogs each day, you need to find someone to do the walking with you. In this model, you are still walking dogs, but you have sourced out a local college student who is studying to be a veterinarian to help. You agree to pay them a certain amount, then you can now walk 40 dogs a day. If the winters are too cold for you to personally walk dogs, you find a second employee. Now, potentially, when the weather warms up, you have the ability to walk up to 60 dogs a day, should the need arise. You now have built a viable small business, using the very basic ideas of business growth that America was founded on and that we have discussed in this book. Oh, yeah, and you did it because you believed in yourself.

This all began with the idea of empowerment, then it moved on to finding something you could do, some widget that you could utilize to build a business. The owner of this business now can protect what he has built with his or her offensive line, and as the business grows, that person is no longer "tied" to walking dogs. They may choose to do so, but now they are managing a business that effectively runs without them. Should they have a medical setback, the business will still generate revenue. They have protected themselves from many of the setbacks that, in another life, could have proven financially devastating. That is what this book is all about.

About the Author

Melinda Curle was diagnosed with Juvenile Myoclonic Epilepsy at the age of 13. Growing up near Washington, D.C. inspired her to pursue her Bachelor's Degree in Political Science and work on Capitol Hill as a staffer. After struggling with employment and health for years, she began taking an active role in her health and wellness and has been successful in mitigating the role that epilepsy plays in her life. Successfully completing her Masters in Special Education, she then taught middle- and high-school children with learning disabilities for several years. She began to realize that her passion was not just teaching, but helping to improve her life and the lives of others. She has shared that story here and her first book, Seizure Free – Addressing the Causes of Seizure Naturally. She shares her home in Virginia with an old mutt named Charlie.

Melinda Curle is available for epilepsy empowerment coaching. You can contact her through her blog, **melindacurle.com.** Go to her website today and sign up for her brain foods ebook to find some healthy and delicious brain boosting recipes.

More Books From Perfect Publishing

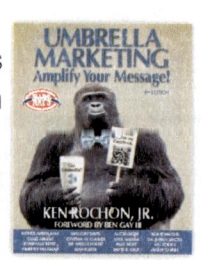

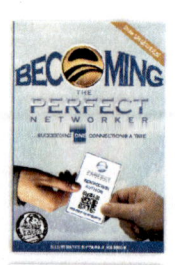

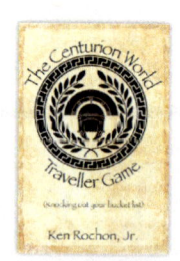

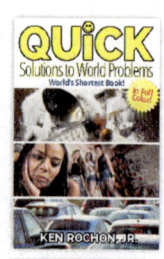

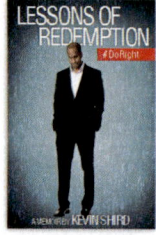

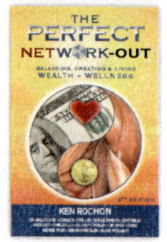

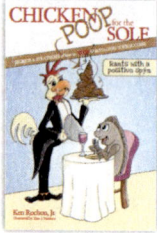

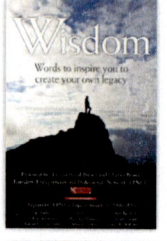

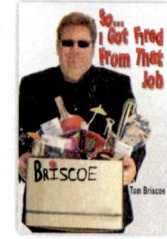

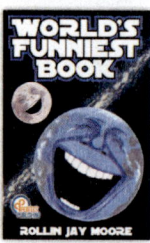

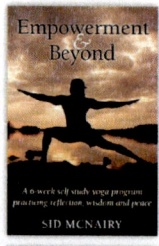

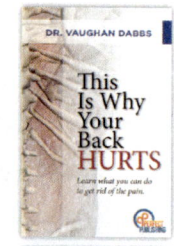

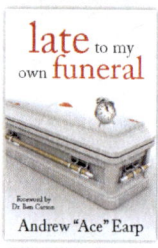

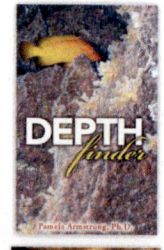

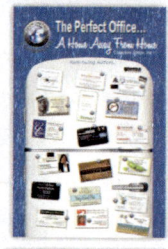

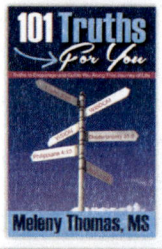

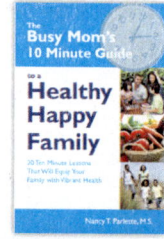

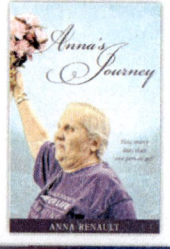

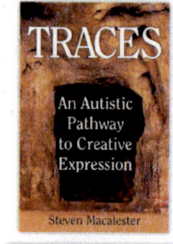

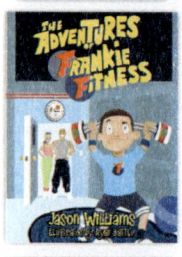

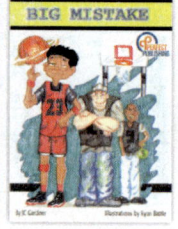

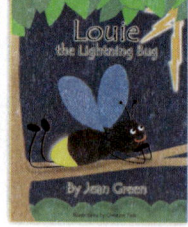

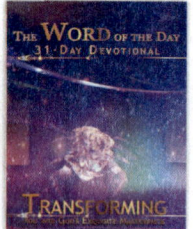

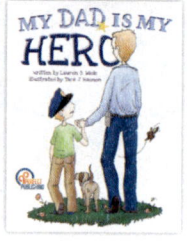

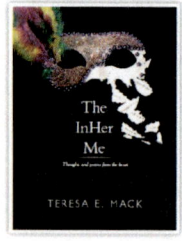

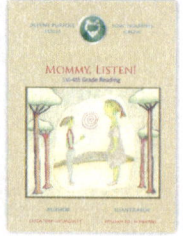

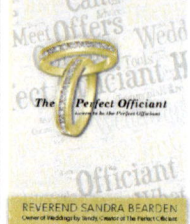

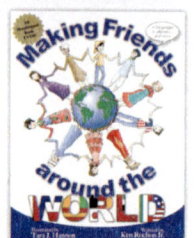

www.PerfectPublishing.me